SMART NURSE

A Guide For First Time Nurses

Table Of Contents

Table Of Contents 2

Introduction 3

CHAPTER ONE: Your First Day 8

CHAPTER TWO: Meeting the Team 28

CHAPTER THREE: Dealing with Death 56

CHAPTER FOUR: How To Choose Your Field And A Hospital. 82

CHAPTER FIVE: Ways To Make Extra Cash 110

CHAPTER SIX: Career management: life after nursing 135

CHAPTER SEVEN: Handling Sensitive Issues 161

Introduction

There is no crime in being a novice, in fact when you utilize your "rookie stage" it helps you to avoid the same mistakes your "predecessors" have fallen into. When we do things for the first time, we are new in the system and in-experienced, but that doesn't mean we are as blank as a piece of paper and we could be easily swayed, No! What we have that others don't have is that we have the opportunity to make things better, do things better and enjoy improved advantages of our own success and a joint one too. Being a nurse is not a day's job neither is it a Herculean task too. As a professional nurse, you have passed through several stages of education and training at the nursing school or any nursing training center. But what may be new to you now is your *first day as a nurse*. And that is the essence of this book.

First I would like to congratulate for accepting the call to be a nurse. Yes, it's a calling! More of something ministerial to me. I would like you to take your time to say the Nightingale Pledge:

I solemnly pledge myself before the almighty and in the presence of this assembly,

To pass my life in purity and to practice my profession faithfully. I will

Abstain from whatever is deleterious and mischievous, and will not

Take or knowingly administer any harmful drug. I will do all in my power

To maintain and elevate the standard of my profession, and will hold in confidence

All personal matters committed to my keeping and all family affairs coming to me

Knowledge in the practice of my calling. With loyalty will I endeavor to aid the physician, in his work

And devote myself to the welfare of those committed to my care.

(Source: Composed by Lystra Gretter in 1893)

You can say yours. What is the need of this? You may ask, but I want you to be a witness to yourself. Nursing is more than just any job; it is a specialized career which requires more than enough commitment. The kind of commitment which can be equated to that you have with your spouse. Nursing defined by the ANA (2010c), is "the protection, promotion, and optimization of health and abilities, prevention of illness and injury, alleviation of suffering through the diagnosis and treatment of human response, and advocacy in the care of individuals, families, communities and populations" (p. 10). That should tell you what nursing is.

Although, I am not here to explain how important nursing is, the history of nursing, and all other academic contents which you must have learnt in nursing school, I feel that you should take some few minutes to ruminate on the importance of nursing. First start by asking yourself; "How did I come about choosing nursing as a career?" Then ponder on the importance of nursing and how you intend to affect the society with it. Something you must have been doing already. As a student, when you approach your first nursing job after graduation, you may tend to experience *reality shock*. This book is written so that you can be able to control that to your benefit.

The aim of this book is to provide you with enough information which you would utilize on your "first day" and other days to come. This book is to serve as a handbook for you. It is also structured in a way that it uses a little to explain the majority. As you must have noticed that there are only seven chapters in this book, there is more to nursing than just seven chapters, but this is a compendium of the essentials you need as a first-time nurse. Experience, they say is the best teacher but to me it is one of the best teachers, your experience would complement this book. Remember that nursing as a profession has a social agreement (contract) with the society as described in Nursing's *Social Policy Statement* (ANA, 2010c): "The authority for the practice of professional nursing is based on a social contract that acknowledges professional rights and responsibilities as well as mechanisms for accountability" (p. 6). Treat this contract like a contract.

I have also tried to make this book as practical as possible because it is a guidebook. Having said that, I have introduced a short segment in each chapter which are randomly placed. I refer to this segment as the "quick questions/quick answer" segment. You can write inside the book, or you can jot down your observations as well as answers to the questions. I hope you enjoy all the benefits this guide book provides.

CHAPTER ONE

Your First Day

"Our job as nurses is to cushion the sorrow and celebrate the job, every day, while we are just doing our jobs".

- Christine Belle

Recall your first day in High school, how was it? Well some of us may not have the "best" of relationships or experience when that day arrived. But we all had a degree of anxiety one day or the other. Your first day as a nurse doesn't really have to be like your first day in High school or college, it has to be better than that. This book is not going to tell you how to erase anxiety, although I could tell you that along the way. But this book is to prepare you for all possible events that you may face when the deal day comes.

This chapter is divided into four sections; satisfactions of being a nurse, being close to work, getting used to sleep schedule and work life balance. You haven't come all this way just to freak out on your first day, you are a professional, and you should act like one. Apart from the fact that you think that you have learnt all what is required as a professional nurse, you may also be thinking that a guide book like this may not come too handy. Well, you only have two things in mind then-one, you believe the nursing life is an adventurous one and you just want to jump into it, unprepared and get anything that comes your way or you just trust your experience to take you all the way. Your struggle as a professional (not only in the nursing profession) is to execute your service in such a way that you begin to gain respect from other professionals and ensure good working conditions as well as maintaining an adequate pay too. It's so painful that it was well into the twentieth century before nurses, (people who most of the time have always delivered care in hospitals) were given the respect and better working condition they deserve.

Your first day should be the best. Yes! Most of the time it is, we have longed for this, we have studied hard for this, burning the night candle, struggling to be the best, now it's time.

Satisfaction of being a nurse

When we are talking about satisfaction of being a nurse, we are also indirectly discussing about job satisfaction. We should understand what job satisfaction is. After all, nursing is our job, it's our profession. Job satisfaction can be described as an employee's effectual response to a job, based on associating visible results with expected or desired results and is a multifaceted make-up of the extrinsic and intrinsic job elements. While we may name items like salary and benefits under extrinsic factors, because they are tangible aspects of the job, we name other items like personal and professional development, opportunities and even recognition as intrinsic factors. Are you satisfied to being a nurse?

Quick Questions/Quick Answers

- ❖ Why did you decide to become a Nurse?

- ❖ Have you ever thought of any other occupation or profession in case nursing doesn't work out?

❖ In case you are not provided with the best working condition, what would be your attitude towards work?

It would be advisable for you to give sincere answers to the questions above. You would not want to end up deceiving yourself.

According to research, Nurses in Chinese hospitals who have better work environments have infinitesimal odds of job dissatisfaction. Also, it has been tested and proven that hospitals with staff's or personnel's who are satisfied with their current position render quality patient care and patients in such hospitals are very likely to be contented with the services they receive as well as nursing communications too. Patients are even happy to recommend such hospitals. From a particular study which consisted of 20 nurses from a university hospital, the following are their opinions when it comes to job satisfaction:

"One stressful aspect of my profession which affects me sourly is the issue of lack of clarity which engulfs

our function. I think that it is very frustrating, because our role lacks clarity."

"I love my profession. Most times, in the evening, I go home, asking myself; "how many patients told me thanks today? Thanks, or I'm thankful to God" this makes me happy and the difficulties of my profession would suddenly skip my memory"

"At first my job satisfaction was very high, maybe because I was in-experienced but now it is decreased"

"The nursing management is not so effective, I think. They rarely appreciate us for our good works and occasionally they are not fair in their decisions."

"I'm a nurse with a postgraduate degree in nursing. But I would advise others coming after me who have high school degree to further their education in nursing. I may not understand why the education level of nurses is not important, or its importance is not emphasized. My job satisfaction is affected greatly by this inequality."

Note: The above statements are people's experience and the writer wishes no harm from the readers.

It is important you know your priority now, it is also fundamental for you to stick with nursing as a profession, weather you feel it is satisfactory or not. Most times, the job satisfaction of nurses working in a private hospital is always higher than those working in public hospitals. We are going to discuss about choosing hospitals as the book goes on.

As a nurse, your point of satisfaction should be the joy derived from helping people, the joy derived from saving lives, administering jobs, helping the doctor and treating others. The extrinsic values should not be what motivates you, they should be side attractions. Instead the intrinsic values should be upheld.

The following are some factors which affects satisfaction as well as dissatisfaction too.

1. Working/Professional environment; for nurses who sense that their job working environment is stressful, a sense of dissatisfaction comes and if something is not done to make it right, it stays there. It should be noted that the practice of nursing is environmentally significant and this is a major factor when it comes to job satisfaction

2. Having adequate resources; Resources here is not only medical instruments which are expected to be in a hospital or clinic, Human resources could also be in-adequate. Especially when it comes to providing patient with registered nurses. Remember the research we mentioned and the statements which accompanied it? Educational differences are also a factor that could eliminate satisfaction.
3. Ratings of Quality nurses; this is an extension of the second part of the above point. Now ask yourself, why is it that nurses in private hospitals seem to be satisfied with their jobs than those in public hospitals? Is it because they receive fat-salaries, sometimes even the amount the private nurses receive could be more than that of a nurse working in a public hospital.
4. But what do those in the private hospital enjoy? And those in public fail to possess.

Work-Life balance

For so many years, this point has been very critical when it comes to being employed and simultaneously playing the post you were in the family before you got the job. On and on, people have found it hard to really balance work and life (your real-self when you are not in the hospital/clinic) without giving one predominance over the other. Work-life balance has to do with controlling stress, before it controls you, avoiding burnout, making use of stress management and getting the best from life. Work-life balance also has to do with the way your shift (morning or night) affects your sleep, much of it we will discuss. We would leave the aspect of the work here for now and focus on dealing with balancing your life, caring for yourself just as you care for others. Even though caring for others is the main focus of nursing, while caring for others, you may drain yourself. You may tend to discover as you continue in your practice that you are always tired after a long day in the clinic or hospital. It is normal and this is when stress sets in. Don't let it surprise you that sometimes, the stress may not disappear, in fact they could multiply as you go on in your nursing experience but the need to make a life from yourself (personal life) could propel you to another level of expertise.

Finding a balance between work and life is also very important, because it allows to be aware of *burnout* and how it can be controlled. What is burnout?

According to Garret & McDaniel 2001 p. 92. Burnout is a "syndrome manifested by emotional exhaustion, depersonalization, and reduced personal accomplishments; it commonly occurs in professions like nursing" Finding a balance between work and life means stating the requirements, the demands of work weighed mutually to create an evenhanded share of time that permits for work to be carried out effectively, professionally and a professional's personal life to get noticed without one negatively affecting the other. You should know that if *burnouts* are not treated, they could affect the nurse physically and psychologically. Physically, symptoms such as abdominal complaints, irritability, headaches etc. can come in while looking at the psychological sense, you may be experiencing something like anger, isolation, depression etc. all coming from high level of stress and not balancing work and life. A natural way your system helps you to cope with stress is this: the hormones, adrenaline and cortisol, would trigger the body to react and then they alert the nervous, cardiovascular, endocrine and immune systems. But this would only last if we consciously deal with it psychologically. Personally, I believe that dealing with matters psychologically is a strong way to affect the physical.

Quick Questions/ Quick Answers

- ❖ Speculate the number of hours you can work as a nurse without experiencing stress when you are through

  _____
  _____

- ❖ How where you able to handle stress when you were in nursing school?

  _____
  _____
  _____

- ❖ At what point in time have you felt so depressed resulting from stress and how have you been able to handle it?

  _____
  _____
  _____

- ❖ What perfect life do you imagine for yourself even as a nurse? This should include goals and achievement of the nursing experience.

_____

_____

_____

When we talk about making a balance between life and work, we would get it all wrong if we fail to understand that as humans we have personal needs and desires, we have dreams which we would want to achieve before we leave the surface of the earth. Most of us even have the intention to leave a legacy for our children. All this has to do with what we want first as a person then as a nurse. Although both lives are not expected to separate. You should have a personal schedule, it shouldn't be work! Work! And work!

Below are some ways to eliminate stress and to balance work and life.

- Recognize the kind of life you want and go after it.
- Care for yourself by getting appropriate amount of exercise, good sleep and eating a healthy diet. It is advisable that as a nurse, you should watch excessive use of caffeine. Just having a cup of coffee every morning could be very harmful.

- Make use of humor; listen to jokes, laugh. Definitely there must be a hilarious personality in the hospital, make friends with them.
- When you are faced with a problem, you should concentrate on what is happening rather than what might happen. This means that you should concentrate on resolving the issues at hand rather than the "consequences" if all goes wrong.
- You should not run away from problems, confront them. Use them as opportunity to test your secret skills.
- Each day, you should set aside a time when you would think and be productive.
- Take breaks.
- Always ask questions when you are confused and seek for help. Seeking for help does not mean that you are dumb or weak, it shows that you are strong and very intelligent.
- Make a schedule for yourself and follow it.
- I would advise that you should have personal goals for a week. Goals that have to do with your personal life and achieve them. For example, you may decide to have a garden and keep it.

- Don't deprive yourself of life's best: visit the cinema, go out with your spouse, your free time should be used effectively.
- You should develop a "stress management" time-table.

A stress management timetable is a list I would like you to make. It's not much of a timetable but something that reminds you of the past and affects the present.

How you can make your personal stress time table.

You get a note-pad or a diary then make two columns. On the left-hand side, you write things peculiar to you which lead to stress and then on the other side you write down solutions, especially those that have been working for you for years. With this "time-table" you can be able to monitor yourself and get the best out of every experience you are facing.

Getting Used To Sleep Schedule

When it comes to a job or a profession which has to do with late night shifts, the role of a sleep schedule cannot be overlooked. Studies speculate that average sleep durations have diminished from 9 hours in 1910 to as tiny as 6.9 hours on workdays in 2002. What does this suggest, people are not sleeping anymore! Now what is trending is sleeping longer on weekends because they are work-free days. As a nurse, you should be prepared to utilize a sleeping schedule or else be ready to face the disadvantages of a bad sleeping habit. It is very painful that an early objective study discloses that night shift workers attain 1-4 hours less sleep. If care is not taken, you may fall under this category.

As essential as it sounds, sleep is a very important requirement for all humans and animals. Sleeping is a time when the body and mind regenerates and rejuvenate. Surely, fatigue can negatively disturb the quality of performance and health of nurses and this can tell on the health of the patient when it comes to patient care. It is reported that up to 20% of Americans get less than 6 hours sleep on average, nurses and "shift" workers make up 14%. When you stay awake in the night you beat nature! Because our bodies are programmed in such a way that when it is dark, our internal rhythm goes to rest. It is natural and would continue like that. But something I like about nature is that she balances all by herself. Whether you like it or not the number of hours you have deprived yourself of would surely catch up with you and you may not like it. The factors contributing to an epileptic sleeping habit or insufficient sleep could be grouped into two:

1. Behavioral factors
2. External factors

The behavioral factors may include: dietary choices, lack of exercise, caffeine and other stimulants. Behavioral factors have to do with attitudes/ traits which have become part of us and affects our sleeping habit.

The external factors most of the time cannot be controlled: temperature and light, stress and family obligations, work schedules, traffic or other nose etc. are just a tiny part from the big well of external factors which negatively affect our sleeping habit.

Quick Questions/ Quick Answers

❖ Do you enjoy staying up late in the night? Give reasons

_____
_____
_____

❖ Do you make use of sleeping pills?

_____

_____

❖ List external and behavioral factors that affects your sleeping habit and provide solutions on how to control them.

_____

_____

_____

_____

_____

Below I would like to share with you 10 tips for getting better sleep even as a Night-Shift Nurse.

- Make sure your sleep is a priority: You are aware that sleep is very important for your overall good health, make it important.
- You should have a constant sleeping schedule: you should make it a priority to go to bed at the same time and wake up at the same time too. We are going to discuss more about sleeping schedule as the chapter continues.
- Embrace darkness: Make your bedroom as dark as possible, it helps to accelerate the "sleepy mind".

- Don't over stimulate your brain: stimulating your brain comes from staring at screens, taking much of caffeine and sleeping pills too. Control all these factors and you would have a better sleep.
- Don't forget to take a nap whenever you have the time: sometimes, you may just feel tired and the need to lie down for some minutes could overshadow you. Give in to it, you can rest for 30 minutes to 40 minutes a day. This helps you to feel refreshed but make sure you don't nap more than two hours because it may make you groggy.
- Maintain a cool room which promotes a more restful sleep.
- Have healthy eating habits: Don't take heavy food when you are about sleeping. Avoid rich, spicy food or any food which could cause a negative reaction before you sleep. And don't forget your dinner, don't go to bed hungry.
- Keep the noise out: Make sure you put out disturbing noise which may affect your sleep. Switching off your phone and telling your family and friends that you don't want to be disturbed is also a good way to utilize the little time you have for sleep.

- Avoid forcing yourself to stay awake: Adopting any strategy for staying awake for the complete 12 hours you have for your night shift is dangerous to your health. Even during your shift, there is every tendency you are going to sleep at least for some minutes, don't force yourself to stay awake.
- Have a functioning social life: When you are on a night shift, you could get your phone and enjoy night "chatting" if you can. Make sure you have good plans and activities with friends and family.

As much as the societal demands affect our lifestyle and contributes to sleep deprivation, our personal lives also play an active part. You may have the feeling that as a nurse, the demand for quality health service is high and you must be able to meet it. Yes! You're right but a sick person cannot administer any medical treatment. What can be done when it is inevitable for us to deprive ourselves of sleep? Discuss with administrators about ways improvement can be made when it comes to the sleep health of personnel's in the clinic or hospital.

Having a Sleeping Schedule

A sleeping schedule should mirror your work schedule throughout the week. It's not one big plan or time table.

Example

6:00-7:00 am. Wake up, prepare for work

7:00 am -7:00 pm Working hours

7:00 pm – 8:00pm Dinner /preparation for work

8:00pm – 5:45 am Sleep.

For Night-shift.

7:00 am. -8:00 am Wake up, breakfast

8:00 am -10:30 am. Go for a walk or take part in any social activity

10:30 am – 5:00 Pm. Sleep and get ready for work. After waking.

Note that you may wake up before that time, don't deprive yourself of good sleep.

Be Close to Work

Being close to work does not really mean being close to the hospital or clinic you work, no, it has to do with being a nurse all the time. You have taken an oath to always render your services to humanity, you should not break it. Be eager to work, take your profession like your destiny.

Case Study

In this section you are to write or discuss strong points which have been mentioned in the chapter.

- Taking into consideration for a week, how can you monitor you sleeping habit and time management positively?
- Write a two-page essay on the topic "The satisfaction I derive as a nurse"
- When you begin your nursing, experience notice the things (policies, lifestyle) that are "new to you" and how they have affected you.

CHAPTER TWO

Meeting the Team

"Coming together is a beginning. Keeping together is progress. Working together is success."

-Henry Ford

Like any institution on the surface of the earth, an entity cannot do all the work. Even in factories with several machines which could replace humans, there is still need for several operators and technicians. A tree cannot make a forest, you can't do it all alone. As a nurse, you are part of a synergy that cannot be broken. You play a vital role when it comes to achieving the goal of a medical center or hospital. And what is the goal of every health institution? You should be able to give an answer. When we talk about meeting a team, we are talking about making our way into a particular system. A system that maximizes the health and the well-being of yourself as a nurse, quality patient/client accomplishment and societal results which are the fruits of your work. In this team work concept, we are going to talk about the organizational level of the hospital or clinic. The organizational social factors too which are related to the culture, values and climate of a particular society would not be left out. Stability in communication. Which is a fundamental requirement to relate with others.

In this chapter we will talk about management relations. How to show respect as well as dealing with policies at work. You are to relate to everyone with respect, having full knowledge of the position they occupy, and even though you are higher than some of the staff in the hospital and clinic, you should show them respect. Working with everyone and working for everyone should be your goal. What happens in the health sector is that, there is a chain of relation that exist, this chain affects each member and also affects the quality of health services rendered. This chain comprises of the following people:

- **Doctors:** These include the medical students also as well as the physicians. They are the people who have earned the title "doctor".
- **Nurses:** These are the people who play pivotal roles in taking good care of patient in hospital. Nurses are those who sit with the patient, monitor

them, and observe any change in their body. There are different kinds of nurses; certified nursing assistants and licensed practical nurses. They have different roles according to the kind of training they have received and other skills too.

- **Therapist:** They are of different types according to their area of specialization. You can have the physical therapists, the occupational therapist, the speech therapist, the respiratory therapist. Etc. they have full focus on skills and function.
- **Technicians:** Those that fall under this category are the pharmacy technicians, patient care technicians, electroencephalogram technicians, surgical technicians, Radiology technicians, etc.
- **Janitor staff:** These are the people that help in preventing a disease from escalating. They probably have one of the most pivotal jobs in the hospital.
- **Clerical staff**: People in this category are those who work with the administrators in the hospital, they keep records and also help to generate data.
- **Information technology staff**: The IT department help with the electronic health records. Just like any other institution, they rectify anything that has to do with the computer.

- **Food services staff**: These are those who find themselves in the hospital cafeteria and prepare meals, transport them and wash the leftover dishes. People would surely eat, and it must be something tasty and healthy.
- **Environmental services staff:** The electricians, HVAC experts, plumbers etc. falls under this category. The backup generator, water temperature, windows seal and all other building facilities is under their care.
- **Pharmacy staff:** The pharmacy staffs are not to prescribe drugs, but they are to make the jobs prescribed available. The medications are always available because it's their job to do so.

You can see that as a nurse you are at the fore front, close to the doctor and the therapist. You work hand in hand with them. It is important for you to understand the nursing hierarchy at this point in time.

The Nursing Hierarchy

Just like the doctors, nurses also have their hierarchy. As a first time nurse, you should understand that there are various nursing classifications, so that you would not be putting a square peg in a round hole when you're are asking for assistance from someone who specializes in another field of medicine besides the one you want. Now I would provide a quick list of the nursing hierarchical chart.

Chief nursing officer

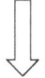

Director of nursing

Nursing manager or nurse supervisor

Advanced practice nurse/clinical specialist

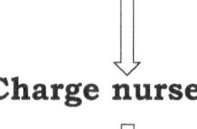

Charge nurse

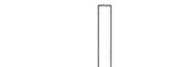

Staff of bedside nurse (RN)

Licensed practical nurse (LVN or LPN)

Unlicensed assistive personnel

Quick Questions/Quick Answers

❖ As a nurse, who would you relate too more with on the staff chain? Give reasons for your answer

_____
_____

❖ What position do you occupy on the nursing hierarchy chart?

_____
_____

❖ What should be your attitude to those below and above you?

_____
_____
_____
_____

❖ Can you explain the chain effect that exist between you and other staff's in the hospital or clinic?

_____
_____
_____
_____

As a nurse, you relate more with the doctor and this would lead to a doctor-nurse relationship. I have not left the gender factor out of this, should in case we have a man-woman relationship or a woman-woman, man-man relationship as the case may be. We should not forget the role of communication in the societal hierarchy. As a nurse, you have to remember that you need to be in the right frame of mind, because it helps keep you in the picture of health. You must have noticed that I have been making use of the word "hierarchy". First let me correct this, in the health system, no-one is higher than the other. We come together for a similar good, some are just more qualified than the other. When you have the right people close to you, success would be easy. Just like a Turkish Proverb says: "No road is long with good company"

The Doctor-Nurse Relationship

The peculiarity that exist between the doctor-nurse relationships is that it is gender based. Most times nurses are usually female while doctors are male. So, it is something like the doctor-nurse, male to female thing. Even though the medical profession is predominantly male-dominated, there has been an augmenting influx of women into medicines. Some years back, looking at the historical background of the traditional doctor-nurse relationship, we found out that; "a good" nurse is someone who cares for the patient by taking care of them in fulfilment of the doctors' orders. While the doctor-nurse relationship likened to husband wife relationship. The doctor-nurse-patient relationship can be said to be husband-wife-child relationship. You should know what is referred to as "the doctor-nurse game". The doctor-nurse game is the idea that nurses were unproblematically subservient to doctors (Stein's article 1967). As a nurse, you are entering a male-dominated profession, as a female physician you must endeavor you achieve the expectations of "the doctor and "the woman".

A small research was made. It includes interviewees of some medical personnel made by the author of this book. This research had to do with the nurse-doctor relationship and it encompasses three main points (1) to what degree do they render assistance in real life situations (2) confidence and respect (3) working with female doctors: does it make the female nurses feel "different"

The degree of assistance

Here is what a female physician has to say about this, mind you she is has been in the surgery field for over a decade.

"Most of the time, when working in an outpatient clinic, who receives a lot of assistance from the nurse? It's the males first before the females. If a nurse is helping me in sewing or something else and subsequently a male works in and asks for a case record, my nurse instantly drops what she is working on and leaves the room to help. I am left all alone"

From the above, we could conclude that gender affects the amount of assistance you receive. Either as a nurse or the amount of assistance you give. Another survey which I am going to give you is that of some Norwegian doctors. One third of the female doctors in this research feel that they obtain little assistance than male counterparts. But we should take into consideration the age difference that exist between them. The interview I mentioned earlier came out with the following results;

40% of the women under 35 years of age reported that they received less help than the males.

29% of the women age range 35 and 44 years of age reported the same as above.

Just 9% of those who are over 55 had the same opinion.

Female Doctor's being "different" at work

Here is what a female anesthesiologist, 45 years of age has to say.

"It could be actually frustrating that I could experience a powerful sense of belonging to nurses than my own colleagues (males). I have kind of "floated" for a while. I have the feeling that it is very difficult because I desire to belong to doctors. But now, it depends on whether or not female colleagues are present. For me

to be a single female anesthesiologist surgeon is not easy at all."

The above doctor has found a feeling of belonging to the nurses' group, she has found a social fellowship which she enjoys every day at work. For her, her relationship with the nurses is uncomplicated compared to that of male doctors around her.

Quick Questions/ Quick Answers

❖ As a female nurse, who would you love to work with more and why? A female doctor or a male one

_____
_____
_____
_____
_____

❖ As a lady, to what extent do you support that the medical society should be dominated by male instead of females?

_____
_____
_____
_____
_____

A female doctor specialist in gynecology, 48 years of age also made this observation:

"The power to execute an order is far from us as a female doctor I surgical department. We don't receive more attention as our male colleagues. The hierarchical system is not in the favor of women. The nurses co-operate in a very aggressive way when they see a female surgeon"

Now let's see what a male surgeon has to say about this. He is 55 years of age.

"The nurses are a competing group, we experience a lot of rivalry between health professions day in day out. Most of them are always directed at the auxiliary nurses. Female doctors could be jovial and very understanding about the women's glitch but a tough disagreement between professions could erupt and they could suffer most when it comes to reality"

Another female gynecologist who is 55 years of age made another observation. According to her, when she was a younger doctor, the nurses assisted the doctor's more than they are doing today. But as a woman she received less help, she had to clean up and do everything herself. She relates that she is now in a position of authority and as a leader in the department, she has everyone under her service. She gets services and she doesn't demand it. You should know that as a nurse, you should give the doctors and every member of staff respect. You should work hand in hand with the doctor, don't let your relationship with other female staff affect the way you relate with him. Below are some tips that you should take into consideration when relating to the doctor.

- When you are calling a doctor, you should have the chart in hand.
- You should make use of the SBAR tool as a guideline of communication. Mainly during telephone conversations.
- You should not begin a phone conversation with "*I am sorry to bother you . . .*"
- As a nurse, you should not complain to the doctor about any other staff.
- In case a doctor's behavior is downgrading, you can counter it by speaking to them privately.
- You should be aware of those doctors who "belittle" you and give them more of respect. It may surprise you that you would provoke the good in them.

- Anticipate challenges even before they happen and try hard to stop them.
- In communicating your key concern or interventions, you should make use of progress notes.
- Appreciate those who treat you well and people who permit a good working relationship to exist also.
- It is advisable for you to add to your qualifications by pursuing a BSN or MSN degree, it fosters respect from other member of staff.

Communication that exist between nurses and doctors affects patient care outcomes. The SBAR tool; provision of the situation (S), background (B), assessment (A) and recommendations (R) is a very effective nurse-doctor communication tool. According to Dixon et al., 2006, p. 380 "communication in the SBAR format allows each field to receive and give important information in a way which satisfies the different communication needs and styles"

Hildegard Peplau (1952, 1991, 1992, and 1997) wrote about five phases of the nurse-patient relationship. To him, these phases focuses on interpersonal interactions and they are therapeutic as well.

- Orientation: This is when the patient tries to get help from people and the nurse renders her help. As a nurse, you are to recognize the problem and offer your assistance to the level they need. This is the beginning of the nurse-patient relationship and it compels everyday people communication, listening, talking, laughing, caring, sharing and reassuring your patient.
- Identification: The relationship that exists between the nurse and the patient should be from an independent, dependent, or interdependent posture. The nurse is expected to reassure the patient that he or she fully comprehends the meaning of his or her position.
- Exploitation: The nurse's services, resources and other things are to be used by the patient to satisfy his or her basic needs.
- Resolution: The nurse is to make sure that the former needs of the patient are resolved and more flavorsome goals emerge.
- Termination: This appears last because it is supposed to be last. It is when the progress of the

patient and nurse is evaluated. They review their time mutually and they end the relationship.

Dealing With Work Policies

As much as there are work policies, there are also professional boundaries. You are a professional and there are some things that are not expected from you. As a nurse you must understand and apply the following concepts of professional boundaries. Now what are professional boundaries? Professional boundaries are the spaces, the gap that should exist between the nurse's power and the patient's susceptibility. An ambience is created in the private information a nurse is knows about a patient and what the patient is aware of about the nurse. A violation of boundaries happens when confusion happens between what the nurse wants and the needs of the patient. Below is a professional behavior illustration.

| UNDER-INVOLVEMENT | THERAPEUTIC RELATIONSHIP | OVER-INVOLVEMENT |

The above can be used to evaluate the behavior of nurses towards patients and can also serve as a check on their behavior. The best kind of relationship that exist in this diagram is a therapeutic one, you are neither under-involving nor over-involving.

From Jones & Bartlett learning (page 60)

Case Study

Elizabeth R. is a 38-year-old woman coming for a breast biopsy into the outpatient surgery center. With her husband, she sits in the waiting room, very nervous, tapping her feet and staring at the wall. A nurse walks up to her to introduce herself and bring her into the operation suite in preparation for surgery.

Nurse: "Mrs. R., I am Lester Nadine, and I will be the nurse working with you today. I can call you . . .?"

Patient: "Hello. Call me Lizzy; that's what my friends call me. Meet my husband Andre."

Nurse: (She shakes hands with the patient and her husband.) "It's wonderful to meet you both. Lizzy, I would like to elucidate in detail what is going to take place today, get some more information from you, and answer any questions you have about the surgery."

Patient: "Oh, thank you. I am so scared. I don't know how I am going to get through this."

Nurse: "It's common to feel nervous about surgery. I am here to assist you all the way today. I will enlighten you as we continue and answer all the questions you and Andre have for me.

Patient: I am very happy that you would be present there. Can Andre come with me?

Nurse: "Yes, of course."

Communication between a nurse and a patient was recorded here and we will see seven good points from what just happened.

In just a few moments, the nurse has achieved a foundational nurse-patient relationship.

- She identified herself by her name.
- She ascertained her credentials and her role.
- Referred to the patient by her selected name.

- Spoke to both patient and husband by their selected names
- She also rendered assistance helping to relieve the patient's anxiety by telling her (the patient) her role as a nurse.
- The nurse reflected and regularized the patient's reaction to surgery.
- Lastly, she acknowledged that the patient might have questions and she was present to help

This therapeutic relationship which has been established forms the foundation of nursing care and a good base for solid communication too.

Quick Questions/ Quick Answers

❖ What is your take on a nurse dating or even marrying a former patient? Is it a sexual misconduct?

_____
_____
_____
_____
_____

- ❖ As a nurse, does a patient consent permits that a sexual relationship should be acceptable?

  _____
  _____
  _____
  _____
  _____

- ❖ If you find yourself in a small community as a nurse, should providing help for neighbors or friends be any problem?

  _____
  _____
  _____
  _____
  _____

Some of the boundaries and professional nursing behavior are listed below. You should understand each one of them properly.

- As a nurse, your responsibility is to demarcate and make limits and margins in personal unprofessional relationship.
- You should scrutinize any boundary crossing that exist, be mindful of its prospective implications and avoid repeating it.

- You should beware of personal relationships with patients who would continue to need nursing services for a long period of time.
- Some variables such as the community, care setting, need and nature of therapy and patient needs also could affect the demarcation of boundaries.
- As a nurse you should work within the therapeutic relationship and nowhere else.
- Actions that surpasses the established boundaries to meet your needs as a nurse should not be encouraged.

There are some signs of unsuitable behavior which may look delicate at first, subsequently they are "red flags" and they should be eliminated:

- Don't discuss any personal issue with a patient
- Do not engage in attitudes that could be referred to as flirting or anything close to that.
- You should not have the feeling that you are the only one who truly grasp any feeling the patient is going through.
- Avoid spending more than enough time with a patient

- Do not speak poorly or badly about your colleagues or working environment.
- Avoid showing favoritism
- You should not meet a patient anywhere apart from the direct patient care setting or at work.
- Do not keep secrets with a patient or for a patient.

Respect

Respect can be said to be something that we give others; it could mean "considerateness" for others and their needs as a personality. Showing respect should be in every interaction and communication. Being polite, telling a person when their loved ones have telephoned, giving appropriate information and being gentle during physical contact and making sure that people are not 'frightened to ring the bell' (Meade 2006).

It could also mean that you don't treat people as objects; you don't speak over, or about, as if they were not present or they are invisible. You should recognize that people have life history that subsisted even before they come to the hospital. The golden rule, 'do unto others, as you would have them do unto you' should be taken seriously and it should be functional between patient and worker, between nurse and doctors. The Bombay Hospital motto, which was gotten from a quote by Mahatma Gandhi, is a very useful declaration you should ponder on

"The patient is the most important person in the hospital. He is not an interruption to our work, he is the purpose of it. He is not an outsider in our hospital, he is a part of it. We are not doing a favor by serving him, he is doing us a favor by giving us an opportunity to do so"

Respect as an unconditional positive regard

Carl Rogers (1961) defined respect or unconditional positive regard as the capability to receive another person's ideology despite your own personal feelings, which may be conflicting to yours. Every patient's reaction to health or illness is peculiar to the kind of person they are. For each patient, the way they react to changes and coping as a patient in the hospital is unique and requires respect as well as acceptance from you. Acceptance in this sense may not be agreement or approval; rather it could be a nonjudgmental sense about what the patient represents and stand for. You goal as nurse is to make the patient have this comfortable feeling. You may come across some patients who have unhealthy habits, such as excessive drinking, smoking etc. which they are not ready to change even under your effort as a nurse, but as a nurse you should respectfully take into recognition the symptoms, values, beliefs and feelings and work with them to improve the goals of care. You should accept people without judging them negatively there by reducing their basic worth.

Ways To Show Respect

You should be familiar with some of these points as we must have mentioned them when we were discussing about the case study.

- Always introduce yourself by name and professional status and don't forget to put on your name tag.
- Demand from patients what they love to be called. Begin formal, (e.g., Mr. Ms., Mrs.) and use the one they accept.
- Patient comfort, privacy and modesty should be arranged by you.
- Don't forget to prepare patients for any procedure that would affect their private space or discomfort. You should prepare them

psychologically for surgery and any other thing which may sound "scary"
- You should demonstrate a desire to listen, help and understand your patients when it comes to communication.

Writing

Now, we are going to deal with establishing a solid relationship. Having understood the pattern written above, you are to provide practical scenario for the following events.

❖ What would you do when: a patient is 20-year-old, a single mother and brings her 2-month-old baby for a series of immunization? Remember, you are a nurse and you work full time in the pediatricians' office.

_____
_____
_____
_____
_____
_____

❖ A 28-year old woman, grava 1 para 0, arrive in the maternity ward in early labor. You are a nurse and you will be with the patient during this shift and tomorrow on the night shift. How would you establish a relationship?

_____
_____
_____
_____
_____
_____
_____

Dealing with love life as a nurse

If you are married, then this is probably easy, make sure you spend enough time with your husband. Even though he understands the requirement that exist in your job, you are to give him the maximum satisfaction when you are not at work. I mentioned earlier that this would be easy if you are married as a nurse but it may sound difficult to those who are single. We talked about having "relationships" with your patients, you can take time to review this. When it comes to your love life, you should make sure that you are not controlled by your love life or you allow what you are feeling presently to control you. This may sound "harsh" but it's the bitter truth. You should know that I am not excusing the fact that you may be "crushing" on any doctor or somebody far from you work place. The truth here is that if you find yourself "crushing" on a doctor, well you know the right thing. Keep it away from your work place. A healthy relationship can exist outside the hospital walls.

The importance of communication between nurses and doctors is also important when it comes to having a love life as a nurse. It may interest you to know that any "green light, or red sign" you show could easily be seen by other members of the hospital staff. It's either this relationship pushes you forward or drives you back. Love like death and suffering is a universal concept (Stickley, & Freshwater, 2002) Love is an emotional state that is typically directed towards others or an object in order to promote well-being (Oord, 2005).

Looking at its effect, love could be said to be an encounter that happens between two different entities. It could be the expression of integration, deep feeling of being, solidarity etc. Naturally, love starts by knowing, understanding and it may lead to personal freedom and development as well as alleviated suffering. (Eriksson, 1990) defines it as a natural human characteristic. This trait changes the human's identity later on into something deep and personal. Love can't be thought as it is not a skill but it is something that can be expressed, something that can be experienced and such experience transforms the human being and opens a new aspect of individual existence and exhibits unexpected opportunities.

It should be noted here, that love here can be agape and not the "real" kind of love you feel towards someone. (Erikson, 1990) A nurse who works in love signals *claritas*, which can be referred to as the strength and light of beauty. As a nurse, the self-sacrificing spirit is given to you by love. According to (Raholm, Lindholm, & Eriksson, 2002) Nurses' display of love to patient can individualistically accelerate the recovery process of the patient, because a suffering patient is in much need of, and more open to, the essence of love. Make sure you exhibit Agape love to your patients and not Eros.

CHAPTER THREE

Dealing with Death

Time rushes towards us with its hospital tray of infinitely varied narcotics, even while it is preparing us for its inevitably fatal operation.

-Tennessee Williams

There are some things in life that are inevitable, some of them may include death. But being prepared for the inevitable can show how we can control our expectations and prepare our minds for what would happen or what we think would happen. I can tell you plainly that no nurse or medical patient is always happy at the loss of his or her patient. As a nursing student you might have learnt how to help family members grieve, but it is very hard for you to say that you have learnt how to manage your personal feelings of loss and sadness.

Here is what a nurse practitioner in Novant Health Kentucky has to say about care and death. "Sometimes, we feel that when people die, it doesn't affect our care, which is totally ridiculous because of *the fact that we are human too."* When looking at the personal feelings of the nurse, when it comes to death, we consider it a part of professionalism for doctors and nurses. I would like you to know this now; when you go through the grieving process, you become healthier! Before we focus on dealing with death, we should talk about grief. Even though it sounds like putting the cart before the horse because after death comes grief, but it still sounds plausible to some extent. Grief can be said to be an unhappy, painful emotive response to a major loss, or death (Buglass, 2010). According to the Merriam Webster Dictionary, it is defined as a deep sadness caused by someone's death. Grief can be experienced by a patient or individual who has a chronic condition and he or she allows that condition affects the quality of life having fully understood that the cure for the illness can't be offered. In one way or the other, grief is affected directly by the person's personality, beliefs, culture and relationship with the departed or the complexity of death. Grief is not something we can hide from and it is not something we can hide either, as a nurse what is expected of you is to keep your calm. At this point in time, you must have been told that you don't shed tears about the loss of a loved one in the presence of the bereaved. More and more of this would be said here and I would want you to take each and every word seriously.

Looking at the temperament of man, some have tendencies to "burst into tears" than the other, speaking of the Sanguine. People who find it hard to hide their feelings under the umbrella of professionalism. Even the Phlegmatic Melancholy's are not left out. They are so sacrificial to the extent that they could blame the death of a patient on themselves and wallow in the pain it provides for the rest of their lives. But something is sure, no-matter who you are, your temperament, whether you are an auxiliary nurse or not, the truth is that we are humans and grief cannot be killed. We can't say we don't grief. It's like saying we are not humans.

In this chapter, we would discuss about grief, how nurses respond to them, the reaction of the patient's family and what can be done. We would also discuss about handling grief pertaining to different age group. The manifestations of grief would not be left out too from this chapter as well as coping strategies.

Please Note: As much as your response to the quick questions and answer section of this book has been very true. I would want you to maintain such standard.

Quick Questions/Quick Answers

- ❖ Have you ever experienced the loss of a loved one or a patient?

  _____
  _____

- ❖ If your answer to the above is yes, in one word, describe your initial reaction

  _____
  _____

- ❖ Does being a professional, means that you should hide your feelings or lock them up somewhere?

  _____
  _____
  _____
  _____
  _____

- ❖ Is grief a normal reaction?

  _____
  _____

Grief

The medical definition of grief could be said to be a normal procedure of responding to loss. Such a kind of loss may be physical (death is a very good example), occupational (loss of job) and social, (divorce or separation). When grief sets in, some emotional reactions would also follow, some of which are anxiety, sadness, guilt and despair. Some visible and physical exhibition of grief can be changes in appetite, sleeping problems, illness etc.

> *"Grief is not a disease or pathology to be cured. Grief is the tangible evidence that we've cared and loved someone"* -Anonymous

We can't say that healthcare as a whole does not require from us a level or degree of multitasking and running from one "solution" to the other with scarcely little time to catch a breath. Passing through the fire of shifts, bed side care, nurses provide help on many levels. This exposes them to being emotionally stabbed as well. As a nurse, all of the time, we happily and joyfully provide post mortem care, we contact the physician, contact the hospital morgue or mortuary. After a patient has left a particular ward or room, next we run into the next situation without having little or no-time at all to reflect on the past on a patient who has just died. Most of the time, any patient who inspires us, we grieve for him/her. We also grieve for their families, taking full cognizance of the fact that an irreplaceable branch had just been cut off from the family tree. *"From the perspective that grief happens, then there is nothing wrong with us when we grieve."* Kumar says. We have established that grief is a part of life and we experience it almost all the time. You should also know that it should not be mistaken that those in the world of medicine are immune to grief. In fact, as a healthcare provider, you need to accept, acknowledge your own personal grief. Freud (1961) reflected that grief is a solitary process, where most of the time, if not all of the time, the entity involved withdraws from the world so that detachment form the departed could be a steady process.

The fact that health professionals such as Doctors, nurses, naively create a relationship with family members as well as patients, gives us a good cause to feel the same sting of the needle of death because we have become family. Any death of a patient can also be said to be a personal loss to a medical practitioner or a professional. Furthermore, unexpected death or young patients could cause the nurse to experience a set-back in his or her belief about life. ICU nurses are faced with end of life situations on a daily basis, as professionals, we understand that death is inevitable, grief cannot be avoided. When talking about grief, we should not forget to mention that it is affected by some extrinsic and intrinsic factors some of which are:

- Level of growth and development of whoever is grieving. A child of age 9 may find it hard to grasp the meaning of death. Even when they are told, they begin to cry uncontrollably
- The relationship that exist between the deceased and the survivor
- The overpowering circumstances engulfing the death.
- Compassion fatigue for the providers.
- Past record of losses
- The medical record of the stayer.
- Previous grieving modes or patterns
- Disposition of the person grieving
- Cultural and social model
- The body outlook

The effects of Grief on Nursing should not be left out too. As this would serve as a guide for us to watch our reactions when the inevitable comes.

(King & Thomas, 2013)-Death experiences can only be comprehended when you study the dying. It is more understood when individuals face their own death or give account of the death experience of another.

Effects of Grief

- **Emotional result/effect**

It is no news that some patients grieve with the family and the patient too. While some "strong" nurses try to avoid any kind of emotional link with the departing patient. Grief can become complicated when it shoots your thinking into a myriad of intrusive thoughts or pictures of the demised. Complicated grief can also result to anger, fear, feeling empty, sadness and helplessness (Smith & Segal, 2014; Brysiewicz & Bhengu, 2000; Papadatou & Bellali, 2002; Tyra & Crocker, 1999).

A research was conducted in the year 2013, it shows that nurses who are under the age of 30 are reported to have high fear of death and are always acting unenthusiastically towards end-of-life care. One thing you have to know is that, the more you are exposed to death, the better it is for you, your anxiety reduces drastically. A study conducted in the year 2010 by Peters et al, stated that: nurses who have participated in a six-hour workshop on dying and death think significantly less of the anxiety that comes with death.

- **Psychological effects**

Too much exposure to traumatic situation may result to mental and physical exhaustion. This exhaustion could dangerously lead to STS (Secondary Traumatic Stress). All these affects the thinking and whatever affects the mind could also affect the physical in the same proportion.

STS could be defined as deleterious emotions and attitudes which someone might experience resulting from exposure to the traumatic experiences of others. (Von Rueden et al., 2010). It could be said to be a state of symptoms that are very similar to those in posttraumatic stress disorder (PTSD) (Jenkins & Warren, 2012). Too much exposure to traumatic events would lead to PTSD in nurses. More also, understanding yourself as a nurse when grief experiences come would help you have good control of symptoms like nightmares, anger, anxiety and depression.

- **Burnout**

Without mentioning burnout, our list of the effect of grief on nursing is incomplete. What is burnout? It is the ineffectual ability to keep up with stress during work hours and this leads to overall decrease in well-being (Poncet et al. 2007). Emotional exhaustion, fatigue, illness, lack of productivity, hopelessness, negative relationship with colleagues and decrease in job performance are all symptoms of burnout. Grief should be well taken care of before it reaches this stage.

- **Compassion Fatigue(CF)**

CF is when your job causes much distress than satisfaction. When you don't feel the "vibe". You don't feel the joy, the fulfilment that wakes you up every morning. You are experiencing low self- motivation. While compassion satisfaction has to do with the accomplishment, the pleasure, the satisfaction you receive from caring for a patient, CF happens when you have low morale and hopelessness. It happens when cynicism and apathy sets in, this can affect your sleep negatively as well as your health. When nurses are constantly exposed to death and they lack a solid coping strategy, mental exhaustion, physical exhaustion and spiritual exhaustion comes to play.

Quick Questions/Quick Answers

❖ What is the difference between grief and morning?

_____
_____
_____
_____
_____

❖ If you feel that there is no difference in the above, state your reasons or propositions below

_____
_____
_____
_____
_____

Types of Grief

- Disenfranchised grief: When people experience a loss that cannot be openly acknowledged, they go through disenfranchised grief.
- Intuitive grief: When a nurse or a bereaved is grieving with a lot of emotions with rich range due to a loss, the person becomes a "feeling griever." A griever who allows his or her emotions push all of it from the mind. Such a person is sensitive to others and self too.
- Anticipatory grief: Cancer patients or people with terminal disease experience this a lot. This has to do with being aware that the day of "reckoning" is coming soon and before it comes, the patient is experiencing death already. It is a preparation for what is going to happen.
- Complicated grief: This is an intense or prolonged grief that comes in the way of the person being able to resume life normally. He is not able to continue with his life before the death occurred.

In case the above question sounds confusing to you, then you just need to know this. Morning encompasses all the methods of learning, coping with loss and grief. You know the definition of grief, connect both.

Bereavement across the Lifespan

This particular section of this chapter is going to speak about bereavement according to the lifespan of the bereaved or the patient. We are going to cover the childhood bereavement, adolescent bereavement and also adult bereavement. Having understood that the age of the patient affects the nurse at he/she's demise, we also need to peep into the obscure future any case of death has to offer.

How nurses tend to grief for Children

Under this section, we are going to describe the grief experience and how it can be managed, we are going to gain a deeper comprehension of the experiences of some nurses to personal grief. Furthermore, we are also going to give a possible insight into the reactions of nurses when it comes to grief and some similar situations. The section of this book has been written from the critical study of eight different registered nurses who have spent most of their professional experience working with a child who sadly has an intellectual disability and has passed on just within seven years. Here we are going to also discuss extensively on four themes which are; helplessness resulting from knowledge and experience, the funeral, the family and lastly concentrating of the positive.

- **Helplessness resulting from little knowledge and experience.**

Two of the eight participant from our study spoke about their inexperience when it comes to dealing with death. One said below:

'I don't usually know what to say at that point to anyone. I used to feel completely inadequate. Most people think of me as the nurse who **knew the child best***, but as his death came closer, I could not but watch him slip into the hands of pain. I could not do anything and I didn't know what anyone else could do.'*

Another nurse exhibited her guilty feeling in response to what she felt as her inability to give help.

'I felt like a waste, I was so useless. I was incapable of relieving his pain, neither was I able to relieve the pain of his family'

Kristjanson *et al* (2010) suggest that the health professionals involved in providing care for any patient during the death and dying of a patient are liable to feel responsible for the kind of death the patient passed through.

- **The family**

Here are some experiences from the eight nurses in our study:

'Contacting his mother by phone became futile after the funeral. This felt a bit awkward, but the feeling that the link I had with her had been broken filled my mind. To be sincere, I couldn't give a solid reason why I contacted her but it was of no benefit to me.'

When a child is being hospitalized or any patient in particular, a relationship between the nurse and the family of the person involved is built. Sadly, at the death of the child, the network that existed between the family and the nurse would be cut off, almost immediately. This experience also has its impact on the nurse as well. Most of the participant in the study complained about how it seemed very difficult to communicate with the family after the demise of the child. It is as if the family wants to cut off anything or person who would make them remember the odd past, but this isn't possible. Contrary to this, Reuben (1996) suggests that what can be so beneficial to the family at this point in time is to know that their child is remembered. And this may result to why the nurse will contact the family after a specifically planned period of time. According to Fisher (1991), Nurses may be actively involved in helping the family express grief and feelings thereby blocking their own expression of grief. As a professional, what should be your primary concern at the time of death of a particular child is the family.

- **The Funeral**

When attending the funeral of a child, nurses have problems trying to "hide" their emotions or looking professional, so, at a point in time they are given little or no go ahead to attend it. But a good cure to this could be-having more work. One of the participants from the study exhibited her regret of not being able to attend the funeral of a child she had cared for:

'Getting an hour off to go to a funeral can only come your way by sheer luck. Even after the fact that you have worked closely with them (the family) when you

have made your way to the funeral, you completely remove yourself and go back to work just ten minutes after.

For some nurses the outsider feeling could not leave them:

'When I attended the funeral, I felt like an outsider just looking in on a family, a unit in which I and other nurses just played our little part.

(Field *et al* 2005) concentrates on the 'continuing bonds' which is directly contrary to closure. In his literature, he states that the continuing bonds are more beneficial to the families than the nurses. In the real sense of it, nurses must continue to provide moral, psychological support to the family before and after the funeral. It the study used in this section, most nurses valued attending the funeral, and this may be because they care about the family and they can have full control over their emotions and still look professional. But attending a child's funeral is your choice, even though it should be important to everyone.

- **Concentrating on the positive**

One of the nurses in the study actually used her experience wisely. She stated that the experience opened her eyes to something new-

'An interest in knowing all I need to know about palliative care and more haunted me after that experience. Ever since then, I have completed a couple of courses in that area.'

This is a good example of focusing on the positive and looking at the bright side of things even though you may find it hard to find one. Here is what another nurse has to say about it;

'What I do now is that I ensure that if a child is dying, there is a nice plan in place to allow the child have a comfortable death. The last memories a child on Earth shouldn't be about suffering and pain.'

Religious conviction can also be seen here from the experience of the eight nurses from the study. Here is what one of them has to say concerning that.

'It is very painful and sad. But I know that children are angels because they are spotless, without sin . . . I remember him sleeping like God's angels. His beauty

was like no other. What I think is that God actually called her that day and her choice to go to him couldn't not be changed by any of us. I pray for her always.'

At times, religion could be a relief and an avenue for looking at the brighter side of things. Fisher (1991) proposed that the need nurses have to join palliative care team comes from the feeling that dying and bereavement has to be managed effectively in other environments, due to the experience they had with a dying child. Even though focusing on palliative care would not help to prevent similar situations from occurring, it would help reduce any potential guilt and build confidence.

Handling challenges that may come your way when it comes to the death of a child is what makes you a professional and you should thrive to focus on the positive. Even though in modern times, death has now been seen as a transformed to an event that most of the time takes place in the home, in the view of the family and others even though as professionals in the health care sector, we witness more death than any other. The role of communication existing between professionals when death is near of a cancer patient cannot be over-emphasized. According to

Robinson (2007) most of the time, family members are confused and scared if a loved-one dies, and they may require information on what to do. At this point in time the nurses' contribution should be very pivotal to the general care they offer. We should not forget the fear factor when it comes to reflecting back on the death of a child. When fear comes into the mind of a nurse, he or she may be afraid of the future and this fear may also affect the behavior of he/she has toward work. Exposure may not be the good way to have control of death, but can currently suppress the feeling that may want to surface when a similar experience happens. Another thing that should be taken into consideration at this point in time is that as a professional, trying to hide from the truth may not be the solution. Especially when it comes to a dying patient. Here is what the wife of Mrs. Brian a professional has to say:

'I could feel that we, as healthcare professionals, which is not expected to be so, where hiding from the truth by avoiding talking about death even though we fully understand that our patient was terminally ill. We focused on trying to 'treat' death instead of providing high quality care in his last days'

The above brings us to another point which we cannot afford to omit. This is the aspect of health professionals not wanting to discuss death. Discussing about death here, doesn't mean repeating the word "die" several times. As a professional nurse, you may find out that sometimes your attitude may want to preclude people from recognizing death as a natural process making it sound as if death is a taboo in the society. Sadly, this may continue until the nurses and other healthcare professionals are free, open to discuss dying and death (Granda-Cameron and Houldin, 2012)

Taking the ICU nurses participants as "specimens" for this particular aspect, we are going to see how "leaving work at work" can be helpful when it comes to dealing with death. The first thing you need to know is that you need to be honest with yourself, create a work balance and find a very strong support system. At this point in time, you should realize when you need to take time away from your "professional" skin and when you should avoid events that may trigger grief.

Here is what participant one had to say:

'Be quick to know when you are starting to get the burned-out feeling, recognize when you are exhausted, tired or emotional. This may not exhibit itself at work, but surely in other areas of life that would happen. You should know the appropriate time to take a break. Taking a time off should not make you feel ashamed. In case you pass through a particular situation very close to your home, you should avoid it for a while.'

Participant 4 also had this to say:

'As a professional, when it comes to dealing with a personal lose, you should make sure you have good support system around you. You should have people you can talk to not lament to. You should be honest with yourself, understand how you feel and embrace it, let it out, let the emotions flow, don't try to hold them back. When it comes to a patient loss, you are to be true to your feeling too, viewing life and death and losing patients also. You should also remember that it is just a matter of time before death would happen. And this is a high stakes game of hot potato you're playing.'

When talking of spirituality, participant 2 has this to say: *'I might say you should seek out a spiritual faith. It may not be Christianity, but having one would definitely help.'*

In the previous chapter, we spoke about keeping professional boundaries, interestingly these professional boundaries may be similar to other qualitative study of grief. That is why a professional nurse who has experience caring for dying patients would put up a strong boundary to maintain professionalism and also to protect herself from negative consequences when it comes to the death of the patient.

Quick Questions/Quick Answers

❖ What is your reaction to the loss of a child who is your patient?

_____
_____
_____
_____
_____

❖ If one of your answers to the above is: depression or burnout. Give detailed steps on how you could eliminate them.

_____
_____
_____
_____
_____
_____
_____

Coping with Death

O'Brien Hump, RN, BSN. A nurse who had been working at a Burn center in Baltimore for close to four years was present when a child of 7 was rushed into the emergency unit and transferred to the burn center, she was the last survivor in a large fire which destroyed her home. O'Brien sat with her while the medical team desperately worked to save the girl. O'Brien sat with her, holding her hand and crying as she was passing away. Some 15 years later, this moment still haunts him as a nurse.

'I remember that I got through that day, but the thought of quitting engulfed me' O'Brien said. In replacement to that, he attended a debriefing and

shared many "tearful hugs" at the halls with colleagues. Speaking with some of his colleagues in the halls, this is what he had to say. *'You can't help it, but to put your emotions aside due to the fact that other patients are waiting for your services.'*

As professionals, we have a feeling that when people die, it doesn't really affect our care, but it does and it affects us psychologically too. Responding to your first death can be getting support from colleagues and supervisors. Some coping strategies are listed below:

- Make use of relaxation therapies like hot bath, to enable you to ease stress that may have been caused by patient death.
- Making use of humor too can be very important. But as much as humor could be used, it should not be used inappropriately. Using humor to deal with loss can sometimes be classified as 'insanity' but you should maintain your 'sanity' when this is happening.
- Talking with co-workers is also another way of coping with Death. Speaking to spouses and family members who are very supportive is very helpful. According to Brunelli; *'The people who*

avoid discussing about it with their co-workers don't really survive in the long term"
- Some hospitals could hold voluntary debriefings especially after difficult deaths.

For O'Brien what seemed to be a turning point in his career which helped him decide not to quit his job, was a thank-you letter he received from the relative of the girl who had died in the burn center while he held her hand.

'Although, we didn't really make any difference (saving her life) but that moment was a big thing to us. She didn't die by herself' Ever since then, I have never allowed a patient " to die alone."

CHAPTER FOUR

How To Choose Your Field And A Hospital

When you find your path, you must not be afraid. You need to have sufficient courage to make mistakes. Disappointment, defeat, and despair are the tools used by the creator to show us the way

-Paulo Coelho, Brida

We can't be so good in everything, it isn't possible. Somehow, our abilities would be concentrated on one aspect than the other. It is true that we may find some aspect of our lives *weird*, not because we want them to be, but because we lack what could make it better. Even in the hospital, we have several divisions. Doctors with different areas of specializations, surgeons, therapist and so on. As a professional nurse, there is more than enough good that exist in choosing one, just one of several different types of nursing careers. One step to this you have probably passed through, and that is when you found what you liked in college and the when you chose the nursing program you can afford. Being interested in a particular field from several different careers in nursing makes you to channel your abilities to one aspect which could make you a specialist in it. The structure of the hospital is like that of a chain working hand in hand with each other, the hospital also follows the rule of division of labor in which there is a break down in the amount of *work* given to each person and continuous use of this rule leads to specialization. For you to prepare yourself to join this chain, you must have an area of specialization except if you are a bed-side nurse. Even the bed-side nurses actually specialize in "bed-side" treatments. Even though we hide the fact that the health-world is competitive, we cannot control how we blend to its strong tide.

It may interest you to know that many colleges have now started to offer nursing programs which cover a wider section than before. Choosing the school, you had to attend also opened you to the benefits of choosing any career you want. But it should be noted that the quality of the program you enroll yourself in is pivotal. And for the mere fact that a college/university has the particular course you are looking for is not really a strong reason for you to enroll yourself in that school. What should be done ideally is that you should find a college having high ranking for nursing programs and also has the program you require and enroll yourself there. Yes, you have your nursing degree! What do you want to do with it? Just as there are so many doctors; oncologist, oculist, gerontologist, etc. so also do we have several types of nursing careers. No matter what you are interested in, you will and would always find a specialization that should keep you very happy with your work. Pediatric nurse could be recommended for those who love children, alternatively geriatrics could be for someone who enjoys helping the elderly ones in his/her community. For some, they may prefer the excitement that comes in helping different kinds of people, the constant rush and working in the emergency room. For some specific ones, they would prefer the traveling nurse; where you would work temporary jobs for great pay and even enjoy living expenses too. From the Adolescent health to Academia, Administration, Aged care, etc. nursing is full of opportunities. The opportunities are just endless, providing enough fields for you to tap into.

This chapter is going to expose you to the different types of nursing jobs that exist, the ones that seem to be "very attractive", the ones that seems to be "less interesting" etc. The role of this chapter in this book is to sensitize you on the varieties that exists in nursing as a profession and the benefits that exist in tapping into what is seemingly perfect for you. We are also going to be checking the roles of nurse at a glance, the role, which is right for you, some real-life stories of nurses who tapped into a good career, what they do and the best bits they are enjoying. We are also going to show you some few steps you can use to step up or progress your career, in case you have the flare of doing more and more. We would provide a list of different fields in the medical-world and their corresponding nursing field. This would give you a rough sketch of what might interest you at the end of the day. We can also help you with sites and names where nursing jobs are advertised in case you may want to check them out.

In this chapter you would find few tips on how to get opportunities that are not advertised as well. Expositions on how you can make a smooth transition from University to your new job would not be left out from this chapter too.

I should sound this note of **warning:** If you are reading this book and you are already engaged in one field or the other, the purpose of this chapter is not to change your mind or thwart your visions from it. If you feel any need to change your career in nursing after reading this chapter, you should search yourself and understand the kind of person you are. Just as I used to say; **be sincere with yourself.** You should not have this kind of thinking after reading this chapter; *"Wow! I didn't know something like this existed in nursing, I am going to go into it now, and it is very easy for me"* Once you have this sudden interest, it may die down if you go into it and the desired result you planned to have is not coming forth.

This chapter would be incomplete if we fail to talk about choosing the right hospital as a nurse. You can't be a square peg in a round hole, you need to fit in into the chain that has existed long before you thought of being a nurse.

Quick Questions/Quick Answers

❖ What field of nursing is your specialty?
_____
_____

❖ To your own understanding, explain your roles in this particular field

_____

❖ If you are opportune to take any program as a nurse, which would it be?

_____

❖ As a nurse, what are your roles generally? With or without your specialty

_____

Nursing Fields that exists

For the sake of being concise and brief, we are going to focus on six main fields of nursing. This doesn't mean that other fields don't exist, yes! They do, but looking at this six could give you a picture of the others.

1. **Adult nursing**: This has to do with treating and caring for adults of all ages (adult age has to be specified here, health wise) with "all types of health conditions". The roles of the adult nurses are to manage countless number of priorities, care, manage, counsel and teach the patient in all aspects. As an adult nurse, your work is to improve the interpersonal skills and quality of the patient. Adult nursing may be based in hospital wards, clinics, community setting or even at home. As an adult nurse, working shift to provide 24-hour care is all inclusive.

The following are your roles as an adult nurse:

- You would become part of a busy, multidisciplinary team which would include radiographers, doctors, physiotherapist and more.
- As an adult nurse, you would be required to use your initiative and to tap into your high level of observation.
- Your role is also to take responsibility for the personal wellbeing of any patient.

- You would also be required to work in a high demanding, fast-changing society.
- And lastly, your role includes considering what is Grade A for the patient and act upon such a decision.

2. **Children's (Pediatric) nursing** - As a pediatric nurse, you treat and care for children. You also care for young people from age 18 downwards. Wide range of conditions could present itself in the body system of the children and you must be ready to attack each situation differently. Children care includes babies who are born prematurely, caring for teenagers who have sustained injuries from accidents and facing life-threatening illnesses. As a child nurse, you are to work in partnership with your patient (young person or child). You would also work with other professionals like; physiotherapist, GPs, language and speech therapists etc. You play a fundamental role in the child's development because health problems do affect children development. It also important for you to know that as a child nurse, you work hand-in-hand with the child's family. A child nurse could work in hospital wards, children intensive care centers,

day care centers, children health clinic and you could also work in the child's home too. This kind of care is rapidly becoming community based.

The following are the roles of a Child nurse

- Having full knowledge and the requirements to comprehend the mind of a child and how to respond to their needs.
- He/she must be able to communicate to the child or young adult without using words.
- He/she must possess the ability to care for someone who is ill and may not be able to express what is wrong because of their age.
- Being able to work with the child's parent effectively.
- He/she must be able to teach the child's parents or care givers what they need to know about taking care of the child and what can be done at any point in time especially when treatment is happening at home.
3. **Learning disability nursing** - As a learning disability nurse, you work with the patient as well as his parents and family very often. Your main job is to provide special healthcare to someone who has learning disabilities. You are to help

them to pursue and possess a fulfilling life. Helping your patient to lead a more independent, healthy life should be your priority. Your patient should be able to relate to others on a very equal term. This kind of nursing field is delivered in the adult education setting, residential setting, and community centers setting as well as the house of the patient, workplace and schools too. As a learning disability nurse, you work as a team with psychologists, teachers, therapists, GPs and social workers. A 24-hour care may not be needed here but when working in a residential setting, a 24-hour shift care can be provided.

The roles of a Learning disability nurse are as follows

- Dealing patiently and sensitively in achieving excellent interpersonal skills of the patient.
- Having the potential to work in a high-demanding stressful environment. A place where your progress could move at a slow rate some times
- Should be happy and greatly satisfied when your patient can demonstrate confidence relating with people and has gained a new skill.
- He/she must be ready to adapt, flexible measures and be prepared to play as an advocate for the

people he/she supports and to also ensure that they do not suffer from discrimination.
4. **Mental health nursing** - Statistically, as many as one in four people have mental health problem so the work of the mental health nurse is very important. Mental health is no respecter of age and background, so a mental health nurse should be ready to work with anyone. This area is considered as a complex and demanding are. A mental nurse works with psychologists, psychiatrist, GPs and other therapist too. Mental nurse render their services in a community, residential areas/units, prisons, special clinics or the house of the patient. This field provides much satisfaction as well as reward.

The following are the roles of the mental health nurse:

- Delivering patient care and working with the healthcare team with much autonomy.
- A health nurse occasionally faces aggression and sensitive display of emotions of the patients.
- He/she is exposed to chances to focus in areas like alcohol and drug abuse or misuse.

- He/she must have good communication skills and the capability to empathize with others and also have full understanding of their challenges.
5. District nursing (Home Health Nursing) - These are nurses who visit people of all ages, most of the time in their homes. They may have dementia patients, patients with terminal diseases and others with disabilities. Some may be recovering after a long hospital stay. The district nurse work shifts to provide a 24-hour care just like every other nurse. A district nurse must be a qualified and registered nurse. This field is a very rewarding, as it permits you to have a one-to-one relationship with your patient and his family also. This would help you to grow a strong trusting relationship just as you improve the quality of your life.

The following are the roles of a district nurse:

- He/she must visit patients to administer medications and to monitor patient's health.
- Renders help when it comes to the personal hygiene of the patients.
- Having an excellent planning skill so that you can take good care of your patients, since they are

people who would have multiple or very complex medical care needs.
- As a traveling or district nurse, you must be able to have the skill to put people at ease.
- He/she must be able to work as a part of a team. He/she must be ready to be part of social services group, voluntary organization, and even the NHS bodies.
- A district nurse also teaches patient's family members how to carry out little medical procedures in case of any emergency. Administering injections could one of them.

6. General practice nursing

You must have been seeing "GPs" throughout the other nursing field above. GP just simply means "General practice" As a general practice nurse, you assist in surgeries, take primary care of the team which are doctors, nurses, therapists and pharmacists. "Taking care" here doesn't man caring for them as if they are your patients, no, it has to do with providing them with surgical instruments and others in the theater. As a general practice nurse, you may be expected to work flexibly, coming to work in the evening and even during weekends. The role of the general practice nurse increases or reduces according to the ebb of the healthcare services of the society. Being a GP nurse exposes you to different aspects in the health-care world. You could end up running clinics depending on the experience you have gained. As a GP you can work part-time and opportunity to apply for senior position exists.

The following are the roles of general practice nurse:

- Helping out with trivial operations which most of the time are carried out with local anesthetic
- A GP nurse treats small injuries
- They provide help when it comes to family planning and health screening
- As a GP nurse, you are expected to run vaccination programs
- Supervising well woman clinics
- They give help to those who find themselves in care team, observing conditions like diabetes, high blood pressure and high cholesterol

Other fields also include:

- Neonatal nursing: This has to do with the care of newborn babies who unfortunately have been born prematurely and they need specific care for the first months of their life or the results may be tragic.

- Prison nursing: These are nurses who are employed by the prison service to treat those who are imprisoned. Nursing in this place is very challenging because most prisoners have health problems from wrong intake of abusive substances and may also have mental issues too.
- School nursing: Being a school nurse involves working for the total wellbeing of school-age children as well as young people too. These are nurses who work very close with teachers, parents and pupils. They help when it comes to immunization, screening programs, and they could also provide psychological or mental health for a little while.
- Health visiting nursing: These kinds of nurses provide intense community care by working with parents who have new babies. They help in offering advice and support for women who are in-state and keep up with it until the child starts school. Health visiting service is part of the entitlement of all new parents.

Quick Questions/Quick Answers.

❖ Having read about other fields in nursing, have you become indecisive?

_____
_____
_____

_____

❖ Is any of the above field very "appealing" to you? Why is that so?

_____
_____
_____
_____
_____
_____

_____

❖ According to you, what are other duties GP nurses perform which are not listed above?

_____
_____
_____
_____

_____

Below is a table which shows several areas, options of specializations in nursing. Some of them are open to new graduates, while some need further study.

Adolescent health	Academia	Administration	Aged care
Burns nursing	Cancer care (oncology)	Cardiac & Coronary care	Child & Family health
Community nursing	Continence nursing	Corrections health (working with prisoners)	Cosmetic/reconstructive surgery
Emergency nursing	Flight nursing	Gastroenterology	Hematology
Critical care	Diabetes nursing	Disaster relief	Drug & alcohol
HIV & AIDS	Home care	Infectious disease nursing	Intensive care
International aid work	Legal consulting	Management	Mental health
Midwifery	Neonatal intensive care	Neurology	Neurosurgical

Nurse education	Nurse practitioner	Occupational health & safety	Ophthalmic
Orthopedic	Pediatric	Pain management	Palliative care
Perioperative	Practice nursing (With GP)	Rehabilitation	Remote area nursing
Renal (nephrology)	Respiratory	Surgical nursing	School nursing
Sexual health	Sleep disorders	Triage	Transplant nursing
Trauma	Vascular surgery	Women's health	Wound care

(Adapted from: "Your career in nursing making it happen" by written by Mandy White)

Sites where nursing jobs are advertised:

- Nursingjobs.com
- Checking the newspapers

- Gaining employment into international positions: www.ncah.com
- www.careerstafftravelnursing.com
- www.memorialhermann.org
- www.worldwidestaffing.com
- www.holidayresorthealthandhabilitation.com
- www.legalnurse.com
- www.healthcareprostravel.net
- www.wow.com
- jobs.kindred.com
- jobs.communitymedical.org

How to find work opportunities which are not advertised:

- You should be proactive
- As a graduate nurse, you should get to know people that are in the industry
- Gather enough experience, and then
- Be in the right place at the right time when an opportunity comes knocking.

Knowing the Field that is right for you

It is no news that individuals from all walks of life, having different types of health problems rely on professional skills from professionals and nurses too. A huge load of responsibility rests on you when it comes to choosing your field. Having full knowledge of how to handle unexpected outcomes and experiences and enjoying training and support from you colleagues is just a title of what is required from you as nurse. As a nurse you have the freedom to select one or two from different variety of settings you may want to work in. it could be patient's homes, care homes, schools, specialized areas such as prison etc. As a nurse, you can also merge a clinical career in education or research and management. One attribute you must have as a nurse is that you must be able to listen to people and observe their needs and meet them. No matter the working community you find yourself, you need to set this straight. To improve the care, you provide to people you have to be comfortable with what you are doing. If you choose to take on additional responsibility, you should be able to manage both.

Basically, there are four fields of nursing. These four fields are:

- Adult nursing
- Children's (pediatric) nursing
- Learning disabilities nursing

- Mental health nursing

Working with one of these fields makes you to focus on the demands of a particular client group. Now, I would love you to take a look at the four fields above, you have knowledge about them. Which of them interest's you the most? Now I would want you to go back up, read the roles and suggest more roles of the field you chose. Now give some answers to this.

Quick Questions/Quick Answers

❖ What field did you choose from the four above? And why?

_____
_____
_____

_____

❖ Did you have such a field in mind when you were in nursing school? Give reasons for your answers

_____
_____
_____
_____

_____

❖ Is choosing a particular field as a nurse helpful? Why?

❖ Are there disadvantages in focusing all your energies on a particular field in nursing?

Personal experiences of those who got into a role

The first person is Claire Baron. A nurse who specializes in advanced neuroscience. Her entry route was through a degree in adult nursing.

Adult Nursing

While I was in school, I didn't really consider doing a degree, but I considered training and working as a hospital dental nurse. Something I ended up doing for some months. While working as a dental nurse in a hospital I found out that I could achieve more than I can imagine. This propelled me to apply for a degree in adult nursing. Following my qualification, I found myself channeling all my abilities to the adult neurosurgery department. I enjoyed caring for patients with spine or brain injuries. Even though it sounds scary to nurse patients like that but I was enjoying it anyway. There was much to learn and working in that department really made it easy for me.

In my first role, I was thrilled to help establish a nurse-led clinic which was targeting getting the excellent pain relief possible for patients who have long-term leg and back problems. We enjoyed monopoly of our work because we were really the first nurses to start-up something like this in that area at that time. Three years later I was working with the neurosurgery ward. I received a promotion and I was asked to develop a brand-new role. I came up with neuroscience nurse practitioner. I began handling the responsibilities of some doctors and other health professionals. Three years after that, again, I was promoted. This time into advanced neuroscience nurse practitioner. What I do now is to lead a 14-strong team of specialized nurses and I work as the senior manager.

Mental Health Nursing

Second is Christopher Brownie. A Modern matron in the East London NHS Foundation Trust whose entry route was through a nursing diploma.

*I am Christopher Brownie, I resolved to leave my banking career to become a nurse because I have been inspired by the enthusiasm of my cousin. (***Your attitude could serve as an inspiration to others, be of good attitude. Keep up your smiling face, you don't know who is watching you.***) I found my first placement in elderly care very fascinating, I was so interested in the patients and they were very much interested in me too. Even before I completed my diploma, I was having good plans for my career already. I wanted two things, first I wanted to know my patients, two, I wanted a challenging specialty. Mental health kept calling and it was very perfect for me. The nurses don't wear uniforms and the patients love to talk. In my quest to be more exposed to what I am about going into and to acquire much skills, I studied part-time for a nursing degree and I also enrolled in a Master's in Transcultural Psychiatry. This gave me the needed insight into how I could manage and treat mental disorders that are affected* *by ethnic and cultural factors. Furthermore, I had a year in a private hospital working as a unit manager. I made use of the financial management skills I got from working there.*

In two years' time, my skills had helped me to this position. I am a modern matron for a mental health unit and our team comprises of nurses, psychiatrist, and ward managers. Currently my budget is over £2 million. I don't focus on this alone, I give training on mental problems. I was recently chosen as an honorary lecturer at City University. I have previously gave a presentation at a conference hosted by the National Association of Psychiatric Intensive Care Units. The amount of confidence this career has given me cannot be compared with any. **What has been my driving force throughout my career is: maintaining patient focus and getting involved with new admissions.**

Making a smooth transition from University to a new job

Anita's advice

"I avoided applying for nursing jobs even in my final semester. The plan I made for my self was to spend a year travelling overseas with my friend. Sadly, the plan changed. I didn't see it coming and it happened at the last minute, the trip was canceled. When reality dawn on me was when I could not apply for any job in a "large hospital" because it was already late for me. I was left without a job. Then I resolved to getting active rather than being unenthusiastic about my current situation. I made contact with Careers and Employment, then I got an appointment with the career counsellor. We spoke about my options. This was a very good way for me to remain focused and motivated and to pull a plan of action. Luckily, I found a range of opportunities which seemed to be available. Surprisingly I landed a nice graduate nurse position. Accessing the resources of the Careers and Employment Service is a good way for you to seek employment. This service is available for you 12 months after you graduate, so I would advise you to tap into it."

A good transition from university to a new job requires you to prepare your mind psychologically. You should also anticipate some discomfort. This would help you to control any new experience that may come your way. When you changing from the life of a student to that of an employee, you may be thinking of having some "real" things in place, like moving to a house, being independent. Make necessary adjustments according to how it comes, there is no need to rush into the employment world, you still have much time to spend there.

Guide in Choosing a Hospital

In choosing a hospital, there are some things you should consider. First you are not a patient who needs emergency treatment, you are to offer those emergency treatment (if that is what you do). You are a staff and choosing your work place should be very important just as your career is also important. When it comes to choosing a hospital, you must consider the distance that exists between your house and the hospital or clinic. Are you a kind of person who wants his/her work place near or far? Are you psychologically bound to your work place? Remember that whether you are close to the hospital or not, you must be punctual.

Secondly the quality of the hospital. The quality determines the kind of health care they provide. A hospital which provides quality health-care service and also have a functioning field of what you are aiming for should be the best for you. You can find information about hospital quality by visiting "Find and Compare Hospitals" on line.

In conclusion, choosing your field as nurse makes you to be fully committed to a course. It channels your effort to a particular thing and if you follow it effectively, you would become a professional in it. There is no limit for you as a nurse.

CHAPTER FIVE

Ways To Make Extra Cash

Money isn't the most important thing in life, but it's reasonably close to oxygen on the 'gotta have it' scale.

-Zig Ziglar

Why do we work? I would love you to take some time to think about the reason you chose nursing as a profession, but as you do so, think of it as a self-less service. What goes on in your mind right now? I may not be able to say that but I can show you a picture of what you must be thinking right now. Imagine you are earning $1 a year a nurse . . . Now, can you get the picture? No matter how hard we try to hide it, money will and would always be an extrinsic factor which affects our attitude towards some aspects in life. Even though as nurses, we don't render our services to humanity for the money, we help people because we know it is our duty to do so and that is the calling we have received, but the role money plays cannot be placed aside. Apart from the fact that it serves as an external or extrinsic motivation, it also serves as our "achievement" at the long run. Looking at it from the terms of being retired or old age, what can we fall back to, if there is no money? Our retirement scheme is totally built on money and this is very important for our total wellbeing.

The importance of money cannot be over-emphasized as it can be listed into three major reasons: we need money for food, we need money for clothing and lastly for shelter. Elementarily, these are the three basic needs for a successful life and these needs need. Our jobs are what takes care of these needs. Although we can mention at least fifteen reasons why money may not be as important as we say it is, but just as Zig Ziglar says; it is a "gotta have it" entity. You just got to have it, just as oxygen is needed to live, money is also needed to run our day to day life. Money is very essential as it holds a value for things. In a quick study which I conducted out of the "medical world". This includes meeting random people, I asked them a very simple question: Is money important in our daily lives? What I recorded was that 67% answered yes, while 33% answered no.

More importantly, money is needed to stay healthy. And that is why the say "health is wealth". Have thought of turning that statement into "wealth is health" but in this aspect, we would need to start marking a demarcation between those who are known as the "wealthy" and those who are "living". When people get ill, and they don't have enough money, going to the hospital could be very hard. Besides, getting good treatment from the doctors and nurses in the hospital may not be possible. It is no news that the rich make use of money to solve their health problems. With money they could "prevent death". Apart from all these, we need money to raise our living standard.

As a nurse you may claim that job satisfaction and a sense of purpose handles your productivity, salary does that too. Salary is a set wage that is based on the expected duties you are required to perform as a nurse. A base salary is the one you have with security. It must be in accordance to at least the minimum pay. But we should consider our level when it comes to receiving salary. As a registered nurse, you have an edge over others when it comes to getting a reasonable amount of money as your base salary. This may be one of the value of the RN license. In comparison to the LPN (Licensed Practical Nurse) and the LVN (Licensed Vocational Nurse) you earn drastically more. If you belong to either the LVN or the LPN, knowing this may serve as your "inspiration" to further your education and become a RN, but this is just a title of the benefits of being a Registered nurse. The Bureau of Labor statistics propose that the median annual salary of a RN as at 2012 was $65,470. That is not the full stat. there, remember that we used the word "median" so mathematically speaking half of the workers should earn as high as $94, 720 annually. With these numbers, you should have a rough idea of how much your starting salary would be as a RN. For the lower level nurses, people working under the RN, the Bureau of Labor statistics states that their average earnings are within $41,540 or thereabouts. For professionals who are working on a particular field who are collectively referred to as (APRNs) earn a minimum wage of $96,460. As at 2012! I don't know how much it would be now, but something I can be sure of, it increases yearly. Remember that in the previous chapter, we talked about focusing on a particular field, this is one of the benefits you get from following a course.

In this chapter, we are going to be discussing about ways we can make extra cash as a nurse. What I am about to say here shouldn't provoke any negative reaction from you. It is the plain truth and I hope that when you begin to see the salary estimate for some fields as a nurse you wouldn't not nurse the notion to leave where you are because of paper. Money should not serve as a major reason for you to change your field or hospital. Well the real truth is this: if you need more money, you need to study more. This chapter would open your eyes to the salary bracket of different types of nurses. We would also explore the financial advantages in working extra hours and lesser hours too.

Making more money as a traveling Nurse

Becoming a travel nurse opens a gate of financial benefit. Even though it may be hard to calculate the annual income of a travel nurse, they work on contracts. They can work on multiple contracts and each offers different base pay, non-taxable items as well as reimbursements. To get a sketch of the travel nurse's salary, you need to make some little calculations on bits of information which should be provided by your recruiter. Looking below is a blend of all the types of pay in getting the true hourly pay.

$250 a week for meals ×13 weeks	$3,250
$2,000 per month lodging ×3 months	$6,000
$500 travel reimbursement (once)	$500
Total:	$9,750
Divided by the total hours spent working hours	/468
Non-taxable stipend pay for each hour	=$20.83
Adding the base pay:	+$20
Total amount in this blend: per hour	**$40.83**

The travel nurse also enjoys additional benefits such as: receiving payment for housing and living arrangements by the travel nursing agency, taking advantage of tax free reimbursements. The travel nurse also enjoys extension bonuses which are offered at the end of the contract. Some travel nurses can also be offered extended contract as well as a full-time position which leads to additional income.

Looking at it critically, you would notice that when you make a total add up of all the aspect of the travel nurse's salary, you would find out that they are among the highest paid nurses in the medical-world.

Quick Questions/Quick Answers

❖ At what point in time as money become of extrinsic motivation for you as a nurse when choosing your field?

_____
_____
_____

❖ What are the things do you feel money cannot bye and how have they affected your life?

_____
_____
_____
_____
_____
_____

❖ Should medical services be rendered to people who cannot afford it? State how your answer would affect the expenses of the hospital.

_____
_____
_____
_____
_____
_____
_____

Below is a top nursing salary list by career

Nursing Career	Average Annual Salary Range
Ambulatory Care Nurse Salary RN Diploma, ASN or BSN	$66,658-$199,000
Camp Nurse, RN Diploma, ASN or BSN	$31,000 Average
Cardiac Care Nurse ASN or BSN	$60,000-$90,000
Cardiac Cath Lab Nurse ASN or BSN	$82,000-$166,000

Case Management BSN and MSN	$65,000-$84,000
Certified Nurse Midwife BSN and MSN	$87,000- $112,000
Clinical Nurse Leader BSN and MSN	$86,000-$112,000
Clinical Nurse Salary	$86,000-$120,000
Correctional Facility Nurse LPN/LVN	$65,000-$107,000
Dermatology Nurse LPN, ASN, or BSN	$85,000 average
Independent Nurse Contractor RN Diploma, ASN or BSN	$40,000-$70,000
Infection Control Nurse Salary AS N or BSN	$66,000-94,000
Neonatal Intensive Care Nurse RN Diploma, ASN or BSN	$53, 000-$96,000
Neuroscience Nurse RN Diploma, ASN or BSN	$58,000-$100,000

Nephrology Nurse RN Diploma, ASN or BSN	$52, 000-$92,000
Oncology Nurse BSN	$53,000-$83,000
Otorhinolaryngology Nurse RN Diploma, ASN or BSN	$46,000- $93,000
Licensed Practical LPN	$40,000 average
Long Term Care RN Diploma, ASN or BSN	$30,000-$78,000
Travelling nurse pay RN Diploma, ASN or BSN	$50,000-$80,000
School Nurse RN Diploma	$30,000-$75,000
Sub-acute Nurse ASN or BSN	$30,000-$96,000
Psychiatric Nurse BSN and MSN Multifaceted	$74,000-$126,000
Rural Nurse RN Diploma	$48,000-$83,000

If the above list looks attractive to you, well that is just little of what you can get as a nurse. If you don't still have the intention to further your education as a nurse, the above list must have proved a strong point to you.

Making your bank account happy by working extra hours

Quickly, I would like to share with you some ways you can make your bank account happy as a nurse. This part is going to be about working extra hours (extra shifts) and Per Diem shifts.

1. Extra Shifts

In taking an extra shift, you speak to your supervisor or unit clerk. Web-based systems are provided by some hospitals where you can log in and sign for extra shift. Even though this pays, it can be very detrimental to the nurse. Working overtime or taking extra shifts increases your income. But you should be warned that this something you should not do consistently for two weeks. Remember that we have mentioned in this book that depriving yourself of good rest can lead to break down and burn out too.

2. Per Diem Shifts

This is a very fluid and easy kind of shift. "Per diem" literally means "day-by-day". This kind of shift is based on a day to day performance. In some cases, some agencies make this kind of shift very lucrative by giving the nurse his/her pay that day, quickly after he/she has completed the shift.

The following are other ways you can make extra cash as a nurse

- Immunization clinics: Prior to the flu season, it is possible for you get a temporary job administering flu shots. Going through the staffing agencies within your locale is very important. You can visit sites like; www.indeed.com for adverts placed on such positions like this.
- Proffering Medical transcription: medical transcription has to do with transcribing digital voice recordings of dictated medical reports. The beauty about this is that you can work at your own pleasure. What you need is a computer, internet access and time. But something about this is that you need to take some courses and

become certified to do this. That is very easy, you can take course online.
- Teaching CPR and First Aid: The cost to become a certified CPR instructor is minimal. The American Red Cross offers training. You market your services to different boards of education, companies, daycares etc. then wait patiently for a contract from them. You can do this on a part-time interval, apart from getting money, you would be opportune to get another deal from the company that has contacted you. For example, you may offer CPR and First Aid teaching in a school and surprisingly the school doesn't have any school nurse, your services may be needed.
- Call center nursing: In call center nursing, you offer advice to random callers on how they can deal with medical situations. Basically, you perform a telephone triage.

Making money as a missionary Nurse

Who is a missionary nurse? A missionary nurse can be said to be someone who is trained physically and spiritually to meet the needs of the people. Missionary nurses are sent to other countries to render help to those that are in need of urgent medical care. Their work is to treat people who are injured, who are sick and also to share the same faith with them to. The missionary nurses strongly believe in the perfect combo of faith and healing power to effectively heal the people.

In training to become a missionary nurse, you would first become a certified nurse. You are advised to take courses on international health care, as this would be very useful to you. Next, you are to take the NCLEX (National Council Licensure Exam). Even though the process differs according to country to country, as a missionary nurse, you would be expected to follow all the rules of your country. A missionary nurse would also receive seminary education as well as religious education. Advisably, it is important you learn the language of the country which would host you. Most of the time, the missionary nurses make use of their skills in helping out in the third-world countries. Most of them consider it a calling and not a job. They set up clinics, educate patients concerning proper nutrition, they also help in grass root development. As a missionary nurse, you work with nonprofit organizations and churches too. Now, where does the extra income come in? First, I would advise that if you are really "money-minded", missionary nursing may disappoint you. Missionary nurses receive base payments and income from the agency requiring their service. When they get to the country they are sent to, they receive daily incentive as well as income from the citizens over there. Their expenses are reduced as the basic amenities which includes; food, shelter and clothing are provided for them free. It works in two ways, either the missionary nurses are "over paid" or "under paid". Due to geographical changes, it would take high adaptive skills from them to be able to acclimatize their body system with the external changes.

Independent nurse; Independent Income

Long time ago, nurses simply apply for work in a hospital, work the number of hours given to him/her, accept vacation time and would receive a good pay. But today, this is no longer true! It surprising that there is a general shortage of nurses in America. It is estimated that in the next ten years a shortage of 250,000 nurses would occur. However, one would have expected that the continuous influx of people into the medical world would solve this but that is not the case. Nurses fail to take advantage of their own "scarcity". The leverage they possess has eluded them. They have become very comfortable with working in one facility and it may be because they are afraid to lose their benefits. Nurses fail to realize that they are in huge demand. Becoming independent has to do with establishing your own medical staffing agency. What are you going to be doing here? Very easy, you will be providing nurses to others. It is all about understanding the demand and supply forces for nurses in the medical world. For example, you make a $70,000 a year from your personal regular job, you get a registry for three full time nurses and this gives you over $100,000 in net profits-the money with you after you have paid your nurses. It may surprise you with only three full-time nurses you have made more money than your personal full-time job. What may be very hard for you is managing your own nursing registry, and this should be very easy because indirectly you are taking active part in management, especially in the hospital you work. As a nurse you can either work more-gain more money or you work less and still gain more money.

Advanced Registered Nursing Specialties and their income

Below are 11 high paying RN specialties. The beauty about the RN careers is that a multiple career path you can choose from is provided and this usually come with salary increase.

- Certified Nurse Midwife: They receive $85,000 on an average, while they work in OB/Gyn offices, hospitals or clinics. As a certified Midwife nurse, you can choose to open a private institution or decide to work privately on your own.
- Psychiatric Nurse Practitioner: Their total income ranges around $89,624 to $98,456. This position requires someone with a master's degree specialty in psychiatric nursing. They work with the psychiatric physician.
- Family Nurse: the average earnings of an Advanced RN family nurse practitioner are $83,527 per annum. To be a family nurse practitioner (FNP), you must have gotten a special certification in family practice as well as a master's degree. Most of the time, they perform close to the same functions of the doctors. They

assess the patient, prescribe medications and treat them too.
- Pain Management Nurse: These are nurses who help patient manage pains after surgery or when passing through any health crisis. They have advanced credentials and earn up to $90,000 per year.
- Nursing Administrator: This can be referred to as a behind the scene position. When you are an administrator, you oversee other nurses. You also perform HR functions alongside your administrative functions. On an average, they receive $80,351 per annum.
- Certified Registered Nurses Anesthetics (CRNA): This particular RN specialty commands the highest paid $133,000 per year. It is a highly skilled profession as it involves administering and prepping anesthesia to patients. The high income comes with an additional educational requirement. You must have a license from the American Association of Nurse Anesthetist (AANA).
- Clinical nurse Specialist: This requires additional training as well as advanced skills. Becoming a clinical nurse specialist (CNS) means that you

have decided to concentrate on a particular clinic or a unit in a clinic/hospital. They receive a pay of $80,984 per year.

- Nurse Educator: This has to do with working directly with nurses to assist them in having their educational credits. As a RN under this category, you receive $69,294 yearly.
- Gerontological Nurse Practitioner: A certified Gerontological nurse practitioner (CGNP) earns to the tune of $95,070 as at May 2013. Working with the elderly patients could be very easy and lucrative too.
- Neonatal Nurse: The average hourly wage for those taking care of newborn babies is $29.76 per hour. The neonatal intensive care unit could earn you more.
- General Nurse Practitioner: Per year, those in this grouping earn as much as $97,990 as at May 2014. As a GNP you could work independently or with a healthcare team.

I came across the story of Burke Birch and I would like to share it with you.

My sojourn into the health-care world, especially nursing is a very long one...

Not to bore you with the details, I would just tell you directly that I debated on entering the field for close to 5 years. Two times, it was accepted into different schools only for me to abscond at the very last minute because of some reasons. At the end of it, I got a job as a buyer with a large sporting goods store. This sounded like something PERFECT for me, but after the first day, I returned home to lament to my wife that I had taken the wrong option. To make matters worse, the job only paid me $38,000 a year. I and my wife were hoping to have children and this wasn't enough for us.

I traced my steps back and I found myself in nursing school, lucky me, I gain admittance to what seemed to be an accelerated BSN program and I completed it in the year 2013. Before I got into school, I had spent much time making calculations of getting a "reasonable" salary where I lived. What I figured out was that I would be earning around $10,000-$15,000 as a nurse.

My first job as a nurse was in a Level 1 Trauma ICU. And lucky me, I got the job right out of school. I received $23/hour and a base of $41,000. It wasn't much, so I sourced for ways I could make more money. First, I took advantage of the premium my hospital offered for working nights and weekends. I remembered that during my entire first year, I was a nocturnal worker, I worked only in the night and this brought my base pay to $27/hr. I am a married man with two kids, so I don't do the "crazy" on weekends instead I go working too on Friday and Saturday. This raised my average pay for the 3-12 hour shifts to about $31/hour.

So, if you have been following mathematically, here is what we have.

$$\$31/hr \times 36 \text{ hours/week} \times 50 \text{ work weeks/year} = \$55,800$$

This isn't more than $70,000 but I found out that I could get more easily. By staying industrious at work, I got a raise of $1/hr after 6 months. After a year, I had another raise of $1/hr. I also gained $1/hour from preceptor opportunities.

I tapped into the provision of overtime and I was making close to $600-$700 ($50/hr-From multiple bonuses) I did two months of bonus shifts out of 12 months. To you, this sounds as if I am working every time, but that's not true, I have taken 18 days off, *currently. How can this be possible? First if you are to work 3 days per week you can alter your schedule to work for the first 3 days and again in the last 3 days that same week. Next you have 8 days off between your shifts. You can actually plan long vacations with little working of shifts here and there. Even if after I had taken a few extended vacations, I would still have extra PTO stored up for me which I can be able to cash out at the close of the year.*

I was making close to $70,000 a year. In places like CA, WA, NY, $70,000 may sound like peanuts to you, but in a place like Texas the rate at which you can live here in 1/3 % cheaper. According to National Association of Colleges and Employers, what seemed to be the starting pay for a fresh college grad as at 2013 was $44,259. In three years, I got 3 raises and remember that I had raises for every 6 months in total of 9 raises in a year. The amount I was making from the raises accumulated to $5,000 a year. I was making this just as a grad student with 3 years' experience, I hadn't tapped into the offer things like education position, and certification and career ladder gave me. As a nurse, I was making more than the salary of an Engineer because according to NACE website, the starting salary of an engineer was at

$62,000. I made more than that. I was part of the "few" when I said the "few" I meant this: A recent study by NPR has stated that in US, the house hold income is about $52,000 per annum while 80% of all individuals in the United States realize LESS than $70,000

A quick look at the income ladder and you would be surprised at what you see.

Jobs Up And Down The Income Ladder

Income Range	1	2	3	4	5	6	7	8	9	10
$207k+ (99th Percentile)	Physicians	Managers	Chief Executives	Lawyers	Sales Super	Sales	Other	Financial Mana Spec	Accou And Aud	
$103k-$207k (90th-99th)	Managers		Software Developer	Salesper Lawyers	Chief Execut	Sales Superv	IT Profess	Marketing And Ad Mana	Accou And Audit	
$72k-$103k (80th-90th)	Managers	Nurses	IT	Software Develope	Sales Supervis	Primary School Teacher	Sales	Accoun	Polic	
$58k-$72k (70th-80th)	Managers	Primary School Teachers	Nurses	Sales Supervis	Truck Drivers	IT	Accoun	Sales	Secre	
$48k-$58k (60th-70th)	Primary School Teachers	Managers	Truck Drivers	Nurses	Sales Supervisor	Secretar	Accoun	Sales	IT	
$40k-$48k (50th-60th)	Primary School Teachers	Truck Drivers	Managers	Sales Supervisors	Secretaries	Nurses	Custom Servic	Accou	Sales	
$32k-$40k (40th-50th)	Secretaries	Truck Drivers	Sales Supervisors	Primary School Teachers	Managers	Customer Service	Nursing Aides	Clerks	Janito	
$26k-$32k (30th-40th)	Secretaries	Truck Drivers	Sales Supervisors	Nursing Aides	Customer Service	Janitors	Manage	Cooks	Retail Sales Clerks	L
$21k-$26k (20th-30th)	Nursing Aides	Secretaries	Truck Drivers	Cooks	Sales Supervisor	Janitors	Custom Service	Retail Sales Clerks	Labor	C
$12k-$21k		2	3	4	5	6	7	8	9	10

Why do I share all these? As a nurse, and a respecter for division of labor, I totally disagree with the thinking that nursing is a LOW paying job. Yes, we work hard, but there are several ways we nurses make money. What you need to do is to get the right technique, the right system which works for you. I know you may be thinking, is it all about the money? No! But listen, I got a wife and two kids. I work as a nurse not only to affect the world, but to take care of my family.

In conclusion, there are no regrets in choosing nursing as a profession. Countless benefits come your way in being a nurse. Financial benefit is just one of them.

CHAPTER SIX

Career management: life after nursing

"Change in inevitable-except from a vending machine".

- Robert C. Gallagher

Change, they say is inevitable, the fact that we would not be serving as a nurse the rest of our lives means that we really need to prepare for the inevitable. Just like anyone who is working a particular job, either professional or non-professional, the law of diminishing return would set in, the age factor would also come into place. You can't work forever, even if the work provides you with added satisfaction than you can imagine. And that is why there is a strong need for you to prepare yourself for it. You should prepare yourself for retirement as well. There are countless of "retirement" jobs that you can take part with as a retired nurse. Looking at this, I can say it is a great topic, and a topic we need to take seriously.

Talking about retirement we need to consider some things, such as: when do you plan to retire? How your retirement rules affect your retirement plan? Relocating or staying put where you are, etc.

When do you plan to retire? Your retirement date can be mainly based on the review of your social security benefits and all other sources of income as well as your living expenses. Nonetheless, the dates your certifications and license as a nurse has to be renewed, may be a very good yard stick for your retirement date. You may end up not renewing for additional years, but that's up to you. Secondly, in what way does your retirement plan affect your retirement date? Some professions have required mandatory withdrawals at a specific age, and this varies according to the medical institution as well as government policy. If as a nurse, you fail to retire at the stipulated age, you would need to withdraw your retirement funds and this makes paying more income taxes than you can imagine.

More also, you would need qualify for health insurance. You should check if you qualify for Medicare. Most US citizens are suitable for Medicare at age 65. You are expected to sign up within a 3 months window after your 65th birthday, i.e. 3 months after you have celebrated your 65th birthday. You need to be sure that this provision actually covers your employer's health insurance policy. Furthermore, it would be wise of you to ask your employer whether you are in a "tail coverage" or not. A tail coverage often extends insurance when a clinician retires and it covers events that should have happened even before you retire. Tail coverage is not compulsory for all nurses, but it makes good sense to ask if it is applicable and available for you. When thinking of retirement, you should consider the fact that you may have the flare to return to nursing later, not as a working professional but maybe as administrative personnel. In some states, certification agencies give provision for a nurse to put a license or certification on inactive status and a provision for reactivation is also possible. Next you should also think whether you can afford to retire. For example, professional nurses born between1943-1954 should find it very important to look into how much your Social Security will offer you when it comes to your pay when you retire. The full retirement age is 66 years. Once you attain that age, it is possible for you to receive social security benefits and work. You should ask yourself these few questions when you are thinking about your social security:

- Is it possible for you to live on Social Security?
- Stored up in your barns of financial support, do you have enough investments? And social security payments which would make you live comfortably after retirement?
- Is it possible that your employer offers any retirement benefits? If so, you should know when your employer's retirement benefits start.
- Am I employed by the government? Or another entity which is not covered by Social Security.
- In terms of finances, how much would I get through my employer's retirement plan?

Your life after nursing has to do with planning the next phase of your life. You should ask yourself what you are going to do to give your life purpose. It may be that you may want to continue certain professional activities, or you want to manage your own professional organization, have a structured-out plan for the next phase of your life. Doing this should also help you to make plans for retirement by saving money which you may want to use to establish yourself independently. As a person, I love art, and I intend to manage my own art gallery after retirement, I have made preparations for that by saving enough money as a worker. If your interest is getting other light jobs which require extra education and training, you should also have a financial/monetary plan for that too. Coupled with that, you may be thinking of relocating from your former location to a place where you would enjoy the cool air from the trees, or a place that is far away from the hustle and bustle of the intra city. Maybe the suburbs or something. You should have plans for that too. And part of having plans includes, making research on a nice location, as well as making research concerning the tax laws of the state, real estate, as well as rental options for the house you decide to choose. As a person, I feel it should be your personal house.

If all what you want is work, work and more work, but you want to leave the hospital world, here is a quick list of what may interest you:

1. You could do nursing from your home.
2. It is possible for you to get a job in a law office, here you would be taking part in chart auditing

and helping to identify if a particular nurse was negligent and he/she deserves to be sued.
3. You could do management jobs (case managements) and many more.

This chapter is to expose you to the retirement scheme you should have as a nurse, it is also to show you the opportunities that are available for you as a "retired" nurse. We would discuss about career advancement also, in fact all what you need to know about living a fulfilled life after nursing is right here. However, as a person, I feel that you can't stop being a nurse, just as a doctor can't stop being a doctor, nor any medical practitioner can't retire. What I feel is this, a nurse now, is a nurse forever. One way or the other, someday after you must have "retired" the knowledge and skills you have would still beckon to you maybe when an emergency happens or something. Maybe at an accident scene, on the street at home or even in schools, you would use what you have to help the society just as you must have been doing. And I don't think the Nurse Union, or the American Nursing Association is against practicing medicine with a "retired" license. Well the most important thing is that you have saved a life or lives as the case may be.

Quick Questions/Quick Answers

- Have you ever thought of having a retirement plan? If No, why?

  _____
  _____
  _____

  _____

- At what age do you plan to "leave nursing?" and why?

  _____
  _____
  _____

  _____

- Imagine a perfect picture of your day to day live when you are retired. Summarize it below.

  _____
  _____
  _____
  _____
  _____

Below is a quick retirement checklist for RN

- Have you contacted the certification board to ascertain if you have the option for retired registered nurse with the grace to possibly return to work?
- Meet with the board of nursing to ascertain if the option of making your license inactive is available for you and make sure you ask about the procedure for doing so.
- Meet with your malpractice insurer and your soon-to-be-former boss to know whether an "occurrence" or "claims made" policy is possible. If "claims made" is active, you can arrange for "tail" coverage or be well assured that the employer would purchase a tail policy when you get a writing from him.
- After you must have considered the above, you should set a retirement date.
- You should be careful to make sure that the planned date tally's with the date your license would become inactive.
- Tell your employer beforehand that you will be retiring, in doing this, you should show that you comply with any contractual policy required for that notice period.

- In case you may want to retire from affiliated activities, you should inform any committee or the board of chiefs.
- If this is applicable, you should let your patient know that you are leaving.
- You should have a planned celebration to mark your life change.
- It is advisable that you should make a plan for the first day of your retirement.

The Retirement Guide

This retirement guide would provide information on the following:

- Planning for retirement
- Saving for retirement
- Making use of retirement funds before you retire- lump sums and loans
- When and how you should retire
- Making your money last through your retirement- Immediate annuities

Planning for retirement

Just as we have established, the income you have during retirement comes generally from the addition of the social security provisions, employer retirement plans as well as personal savings. What the social security offers is a base layer of protection but that alone is not enough to see you through your life as a retiree. What we can now result to is personal savings and other income from other sources. Whether they are employment provided or not, we don't really want to know that. All these factors joined together is a good motive why we should plan for our retirement, because if we fail to plan, we plan to fail. Retirement is not just for a day, it is not just for a year, it is not just for ten years, it is for the last phase of your life. No-one would wish to die prematurely, so even after we retire, we would love to live for several years.

Saving for retirement

Saving during your working years is as important as working itself. A good way to do this now that you are working is this:

- Have a rough projection of the total retirement income, you are going to need. You can tap into the provision of an online calculator.
- Make a projection or estimate how much are you getting from Social, security and the rest?

- Devise a plan on how to start saving enough for you to make up for the difference.

Saving is very important, and it is a personal thing, you would have to decide the amount that you need to have an adequate retirement. A very good rule of thumb is that you should save 15 percent of your pay for a very long period of time. Now that you are new to the work force/labor market, the best thing for you is to start now. This estimate would depend on some number of factors, some of them include; having a monthly payment for your home mortgage or rent, health insurance, supplement Medicare etc.

Below is a rough sketch of the amount you need to save and the age you need to start saving.

Age when you start saving	% of pay you need to save
25	9.4%
35	13.3%
45	20.4%

55	39.9%

When saving, you can make use of the IRA (Individual Retirement Account). This kind of bank account can be established at your bank or any other financial institution or it may be through a mutual fund company. Having an IRA makes you to receive some benefits, which includes; having income-tax reduction on the amount you put into it, your money begins to grow as tax-deferred and you don't pay any tax which would take your money out, when you are taking the money out, you won't owe any tax, in fact your total investment is tax-free.

Making use of retirement funds before you actually retire-Lump sums and loans

Most saving plans on retirement provides an offer for you to withdraw money on the account of you changing your job or retirement. You should resist the temptation to spend it on things that are not for retirement purposes. A very good rule here is for you to leave your money with the employer's retirement plan or you can roll it into an IRA on the account of you changing jobs. Cashing out the money that you have in a contribution plan would only make you owe income taxes and in most cases, you would be penalized by the IRS on a 10% drawback. Now if looking at the amount you may want to start contributing when you start, you may be tempted to use it "quickly" and may be divide your next salary into two to make up for it, but I tell you that repaying it may not be as easy as you think. Leaving your money there, without touching it, would make it grow into a substantial amount by retirement. You should decide to take an IRA or 401(k) plan before you reach 59 ½ years of age. Any withdrawal before that time would only cause you to owe income tax and a 10% penalty to the IRS.

Leaving an employer with a traditional pension plan enables you to be able to get a lump sum payment. If you roll up this lump sum payments into an IRA, you avoid taxes. And it is very much advisable for you to leave the money where it is.

When and how to retire

Most of us cannot wait to retire. That feeling is very mutual, but when we are thinking about retiring, we should remember that there are some details of how we are going to pay for it. Personally, I would advise that you should retire at the Medicare eligibility age

(65 years). Because if you think of retiring before then, the drugs and the long-term care you may want to receive, would become an enormous expense for you. You should not forget that when you retire, things would not be the way they are some few years back, inflation would have set in, and this would affect the price you used to get things and it would also affect medical care too. We should not forget the pension benefits. You should know all you should know about the pension plan from your employer. In fact, there is no crime asking your employer about the full benefits you get from the pension plan which must have been in place. In case you or your spouse has a working pension plan when you applied for retirement, you would need to make a decision whether the benefits you want should continue to a surviving widow or widower. Take for example, you applied for benefits, your spouse has to give his or her consent to part with survivors' benefits after he or she has signed the statement and understands that the pension benefit will stop immediately, if you are the first person to receive the call of death.

Most of the time, we talk about when to retire but not how to retire. I might have spoken about how to retire some pages back, but I would also tell you that you should leave the medical-world on a good note. Simply put: 'be at peace with all' when you are about to retire. Leave on a good note. In case you are planning to retire early, maybe because you want to have your own medical institution or something of your own, like your own research etc. it is advisable that you should give solid reasons to your employer, why you want to leave. He/she may not require this from you, but it is very important you do so. When you retire early also, as a nurse it affects the patients, be sure to give a very good reason for doing so.

Immediate Annuities: making your money last through retirement

Most of the time, we do think of making our retirement savings last us for 20 to 30 years, but when we live more than that, what happens? Managing your life savings after retirement can be very challenging as you may be faced with many unknowns. What you would need is immediate annuity. The immediate annuities offer a guaranteed income for your life. When you buy this annuity, making a simple payment, the insurance company will grant you a guaranteed lifetime income. Not minding how long you live, you would be paid, it's like getting paid for staying alive. How does that sound? There are two types of immediate annuities, they are:

- Fixed immediate annuities: this requires you to pay a fixed amount each month of the year until your retirement plans come into fulfilment.
- Variable immediate annuities: This plan would also get you paid as long as you live, but the amount would vary based on the amount you choose to invest, just like the stock market. But the higher the amount you invest, the higher you earn.

Generally, the immediate annuities provide diverse payment options. You can decide to choose the payment that has to do with your life alone or you make a choice of receiving payment alongside survivor benefit. So, if it happens that you die before the estimated period . . . let's say five years before that time, your beneficiary will receive the balance of what is left.

You are still very young, and you may not want to consider placing all of your retirement savings into an annuity, but for people who are age 70 or older, it is advisable for you to place all or part if you like in annuity. You should not confuse immediate annuities with deferred annuities. Deferred accumulate funds while you are working primarily.

Quick Questions/Quick Answers

- What are decisions you have made up your mind to take concerning retirement?

  _____
  _____
  _____
  _____
  _____

- Do you intend making money after retirement? How can you do so?

  _____
  _____
  _____
  _____
  _____

- What can you say concerning those who have the notion that planning about retirement is a sign that the nurse is experiencing *burnout* or lack of interest in nursing?

_____

_____

_____

_____

_____

_____

_____

Jobs you can still do as a retired nurse

Now this section, explores a number of jobs you can do as a retired nurse, you should take in into consideration that some of them are age sensitive, i.e. for someone who probably retires at the age of 70 would not be able to take part in some of them. The beauty about this job is that you do them as a part-time nurse or full-time nurse too. But some may require extra training as well as extra degree or qualification.

1. Teach in High school

It is a known fact that nurses are very close to doctors and they are pretty much the next best thing to them. So, when it comes to the knowledge of health and nutrition, they can't be left out. Looking at this, a retired nurse may decide to become a teacher. Definitely, shoe would add value to the quality of education in whatever institution she finds herself or himself. Most of the time, it is not really unheard of that nurses teach health classes in high school, in fact it is quite common. It would be very easy for them because they have the knowledge, they have first-hand experience too with real cases. When it comes to teaching subjects like sex education, they are not left out.

As a retired nurse, this can be very rewarding for you because you don't need to take on fully loaded schedules and you can simultaneously work as a part-time nurse in the school clinic too.

2. Teach basic First Aid Classes

One major thing that nurses learn and have mastered is providing basic life-saving first aid treatment. The nurse can be an emergency doctor. In fact, the nurse is an emergency doctor. This days, a pre-requisite for almost all occupations is that you should know how to administer first aid. This gives a retired nurse a large occupational environment. Teaching basic first aid classes presents itself as one of the great jobs a retired nurse can tap into.

He/she may get to the level of holding seminars, special classes on First Aid and this also means additional income too.

3. Selling medical Equipment

One of the numerous advantages in spending several years in the hospital or clinic is being exposed to medical equipment and Items. As a retired nurse, you can become a dealer in medical supplies. This kind of job is very easy and it is not too time consuming. In fact, you can run your "firm" online from your home. How can you do that? Create a website for the service you render and place adverts online. To increase your market, you can also place adverts physically in newspapers, town boards etc. Sit by your computer or get someone to do so and receive orders. Then the person in charge of transportation, which maybe you also would deliver them to the expected destination. Simple! And as nurse, with the connections and acquaintances you have within hospitals/clinics/health institutions and without, you are bound to succeed.

4. Become a freelance health writer

For a retiree who wants a simple, less stressful side job, the writing world is waiting for you. What do you need to become a writer? A computer (preferably a laptop) and your fingers. The beauty about writing generally, whether you are a health writer or not is that, there is a very large market. First you are good for the job, you are also good in expressing your thoughts and putting them down in words, then what else? Most of the time as a freelance writer, you work with your head and your shoulder. It is possible to contact some companies online who are in need for health writers. If that doesn't interest you, the world is changing now. Having a blog about health and healthcare is something very lucrative. Not to forget the extra cash you would receive from affiliate marketing or AdSense revenue.

5. Become a writer.

Now you may think that I am repeating points, but that's not true. When I mentioned becoming a freelance health writer, I narrowed the writing down to health alone. Becoming a writer here has to do with writing generally. Look up the story of Robin Cook, Francis Bandettini, Lisa Genova etc. you would find something similar about them. Writing is something you can do when you have abundance of time. If you have a flare for fiction, take an online course on writing, go into health-fiction. If that is too demanding, you can provide books on technical topics, you can also publish healthcare books. Writing is more profitable than you can think and like I have mentioned in the previous point, you got all it takes to do it, you got all it takes to make that happen.

6. Run a basic Clinic

Most of the time, we tend to forget that nurses are the next best health-personnel to doctors. When it comes to dealing with patients, bedside care etc. nurses provide all that, naturally. This makes running a basic clinic a very good option for them. Remember we spoke about license being "paused" for a particular period. A retired nurse can "play" his/her license when it comes to running a basic clinic, if the clinic is managed well, in no time. He/she would need a lot of staffs and the clinic would expand. You may just decide to focus on one area when it comes to this. For example, opening a maternity clinic etc.

7. Be a medical company representative.

This job is less known, maybe because it doesn't really sound "attractive" like the others. A retired nurse can be a company's medical representative. Nurses have good relationships with doctors, they are not new to the hospital system and they have first-hand experience with medicines and their properties.

8. Become a Nutritional/lifestyle counsellor

Just like teaching in a high school, writing medical books, a retired nurse has the ability to disseminate useful information when it comes to nutrition and lifestyle. It is no new knowledge that nurses are the only medical personnel's who spends more time with patients. As such they know their needs and every reaction that they exhibit. A retired nurse can work as a lifestyle counsellor, he/she can help people make positive changes in their lives. They can provide counsel on dieting, they can help in rehabilitative exercises, and they can be a nutritional guide. In fact, they can even be a fitness instructor. People who are of age 60 upward should not consider the job of a fitness instructor as an option.

9. Work as a reviewer of Nursing Licensure Exams

This is within the walls of the health-care system but what it more of academics than treatment. We know that to become a full-fledged registered nurse, you need to pass the Licensure exam. Passing this exam shows that you are ready to become a professional. Becoming a reviewer as a retired nurse, comes with a good pay and you are opportune to work with flexible hours. Another advantage of being a professional nurse is that you are exposed to helping a new generation of would-be professional nurses to achieve their dreams.

10.   Doing some moonlighting

What is moonlighting? This is when you go back to the medical work to work as part-time nurse. It can even be possible that you can go back to the hospital you have worked before and still work there again, it all depends on the hospital policy. Moonlighting has to do with covering for colleagues and working some shifts.

11.   Case management.

We would discuss more about this, but let's have some real experiences from Catherine-a retired nurse. This was what she had to say when asked the question: What did you do after nursing?

"This is an important topic. And it is a topic many nurses would have to face at least once in their nursing career. I was a bedside nurse and I did over twenty years in ICU and ER nursing in several hospitals. I was also employed as a travel nurse too. I worked simultaneously as an ICU manager and a same day surgery unit manager. I was also a nursing supervisor for a while. At the end of it all, I was disenchanted. What I considered to be my tolerance was totally breached, then I made a bold but foolish move. I left nursing for nothing and didn't have anything in mind to do.

Luckily, I met a friend who got me into case management. I began handling ethical issues pertaining to nursing than the health issues. I enjoyed working from home and the pay was attractive."

Case management nurses are those who specializes in managing the long-term care plans for patients who are suffering from chronic medical conditions. Generally, they have a particular concentration and a portion of the population of those that are affected. This gives them the opportunity to put more concentration to their job. A case manager can do the following:

- Work in a social work capacity. This may include helping a patient to resolve family financial issues. In fact, they could act as lawyers.
- They act as liaison as well as arranging for transfer within hospitals

As a retired nurse, there are countless side-jobs you can commit yourself to. The key is knowing what you want and getting it. In fact, as a nurse, your work/profession should take all of your life.

CHAPTER SEVEN

Handling Sensitive Issues

It seems essential, in relationships and all tasks, that we concentrate only on what is most significant and important

-Soren Kierkegaard

First, I want to congratulate you on reaching the end of this book. I didn't make provisions for this last chapter at first, but as I began writing, several things just had to find its way to my head, putting it down is problem for me, because as much as I would love it, I don't want this book to be so voluminous. Reading it all through could be a problem if it was so. It is not a mistake that this chapter is titled: "Handling Sensitive Issues" well there are really sensitive issues. As a nurse we come across different aspects of life every day. We meet different people and definitely we going to meet different behaviors too. We relate with others professionally and unprofessionally as the case may be. Outside the hospital, we still carry that responsibility of being a nurse with us to our homes, our families, our friends and even our spouses. Just like any "physical" job, we relate with people on a daily basis and there is every tendency that they "hurt" us or we "hurt" them.

Please Note: The word "hurt" in this chapter is used euphemistically and as such you should read between lines.

As humans, we have emotions, we have feelings. They are things that make us humans. And what makes us humans too is the fact that these emotions or feelings can be affected internally and externally. This chapter is not only meant for dealing with those who "hurt" you or how to forgive. It is all about sensitive issues. I would be touching some sensitive topics which I feel should be discussed. Because the absence of evidence is not the evidence of absence. We cannot just look away and lie to ourselves that these things are not happening. I don't want you to have this "serious" mind, although we are discussing something sensitive, we would talk about it in a light mood. I wouldn't want this book to turn into a horror novel in your hands where you have to hold your breath because you don't know what is coming next.

Things that are written here are so important and they need to be discussed.

For the sake of protecting personal dignity and privacy, I have deliberately omitted the "Quick Questions/Quick Answers" segment from this chapter, let all thinking be done in your head and mind and let all answers be reasoned out within you. Now what are the "sensitive" issues I would love to discuss? Judging from the synonyms of sensitive; confidential, classified, subtle, delicate, you already have an idea, if not several ideas of the things I am about discussing. I have much to say, but I would focus on three major aspects:

- Gender based discrimination
- Conflict Prevention and Management
- Sexual harassment.

Quickly, I would discuss bricfly on the list above.

1. Gender based discrimination: Some years back, nursing was considered as a female's job, maybe because all our mothers have one point or the other played the role of a medical nurse or because of the fact that females are considered to be more caring than their male counterparts.

Well, If you trace the history of nursing, you would find out that it all started as a "woman thing" like the female's association of those who really cared about their families, about their husbands and the community at large. Nowadays, male nurses are very rampant in the health sector. Not only the health sector, generally men are now seen entering into professions that are thought to be unsexed. Even though we feel that males should handle the role of a doctor, well women understand that too as well and that is why they are willing to support a doctor above them, it's just like the father and mother setting. Gender based discrimination could simply mean giving preference to a particular gender while you neglect the other. It also means treating a particular gender more important than the other. When we talk about gender discrimination, we are discussing about a deliberate act of nepotism and favoritism geared towards a particular individual or a group of people on the basis that they are females or males.

2. Conflict prevention and management: Conflict can be said to be a competitive or opposing action

of incompatibles: an antagonistic state or action (as divergent ideas, interests, or persons) (Merriam Webster Dictionary) When it comes to conflict, we are faced with something which in inevitable. It's either you step on people's toes, or people step on your toes. Anyhow that goes, it becomes conflict. Either way, they must have been a deliberate wronging from you or the second party. Conflict here doesn't mean physical assault or something like a banter of words. No! Even though that could exist too. Conflict has to do with a total disagreement between your ideas and that of another, or between your actions and that of another. To some extent, conflict cannot be prevented, but they can be managed. We are social beings, we tend to get angry at people and also make people angry at us. Conflict may exist in several forms: Nurse-Client conflict, Nurse-colleague conflict. Work place conflict etc. Conflict may result from abuse of power within the workplace. Abuse can exist emotionally, verbally, physically and sexually. All these are elements which result to conflict.

3. Sexual harassment: We should not hide the fact that sexual harassment is becoming rampart in

the health sector. In fact, sexual harassment has become a solid factor which can affect the performance of nurses worldwide. Nurses serve as counsellors, but when this happens, who is going to comfort them? Some studies have shown that sexual harassment has been going in some developing countries, especially in the health sector. Sexual harassment attracts a particular stigma even in the nursing field.

Gender Based discrimination

Gender issues exist on the area of equal employment opportunity which excel beyond the national boundaries and it can be very debatable. The focus and the orientation of this chapter has to be determined here. In accordance with some factors that is present in the society, gender based discrimination usually flourishes there. When an organization decides to choose from the applicants for a particular job, the reason for choosing rests behind the fact that they are dealing with other people's productive capacities on different dimensions and it may be hard for them to determine the right one. The attention of some researchers has been focused on the male-female proportion in the workplace being in the goodwill of the male. Some efforts are being made to make sure that there is as system of fairness in the employment system as well as working system. For females to go into a male dominated field, a good environment must be established for them. This may not be the case for the males because they can be stand much difficulty that the females. Even at the high increase of men in nursing today, women have always dominated it and a very few men would try to find their feet (Whewellite, 1987). This high influx of males would leave us asking ourselves: what are the outcomes that resolve from men going into the nursing profession. Is it possible that men are liable to "hit" the invisible glass ceiling of stunted growth in nursing or progress? Is it possible that men would be at disadvantage in this profession? We may not be able to give a direct answer to that. In this study, I would take my time out to go into the implications men face in a West African Country (Ghana)

- In Ghana, men are restricted in their entry into the nursing field
- In terms of work load, male nurses are given more responsibility that females based solely on their gender.

- In terms of equality, female nurses and male nurses are given the same career advancement opportunities.
- Most of the time, male nurses would choose to leave the profession at any point in time in the future.
- In Ghana, it is no news that male nurses are discriminated against in all ways.

Comparing "greener pastures" like the US and UK, the number of male nurses being employed has been reduced. This is because most of them now search for greener pastures to places like the US and UK, leaving their country empty and unattended too. As much as we would like to state it, there is no clear demarcation between the "male dominating jobs" and the "female dominating job" Cox and Cooper (1997) cited the Hansard Society (1990) report that up to 70% of women work in lower level services and sector jobs. In Ghana, the number of women found in the top-level positions were minimal. Looking at the opportunities provided for women to achieve higher positions at their workplace, one can say that it is very rare for women to have that position and to maintain it successfully.

Men in Female-Dominated Professions: most of the time, women who find themselves in the "male-dominated professions" represent the minority, compared to men who are in the "female-dominated professions" there is a "ceiling escalator" men are given all the chances to explore the benefits in whatever position they find themselves. In fact, they could also dominate the "female-dominated profession" and make it theirs. Williams (1989, 1992, 1993, and 1995) maintains that male nurses, elementary school teachers, librarians, social worker etc. are able to ride a 'glass ceiling escalator' moving up to internal career ladders so high that their speed is higher than that of the females. But Williams studies talks about men pushing upward and getting promoted in their profession, he deliberately left out the available factors that the Ghanaian society has. According to Williams, the administrative roles in the "female dominated" jobs are given to males. In fact, men who work in female dominated institutions have very good advantage in career growth and development. In the male dominated profession, the women are handled as subsidiaries to men. All administrative functions are given to them. The women can only get as high as becoming the vice or the deputy. Florence Nightingale was a very strong advocate for both women and nursing and considering the natural traits in women such as: nurturance, gentleness, compassion, empathy, tenderness and selfness give the feminine part domain over nursing. But another question is this; don't men feel the same? Yes, they do, but can we say such trait is dominant in them? It is pathetic that even as the nursing world receives high influx of new members/nurses, there still exist several slots for at least five nurses in a medical center. The inflow of men into nursing is partially driven by the mounting pressures of unemployment. More male employees are very willing to go into new careers, even in the fields that have long been considered as a lady's work. Layoffs could also be a strong reason for moving into female-dominated industries. Child care nursing, which offers more job security in Ghana or anywhere else. Nowadays hospitals now launch staffing drives which are aimed at getting the attention of male nurses, this happens because of the fact that even some hospitals find themselves looking for solutions to their long-term shortage of personnel. (American Hospital Association 2001)

Nursing in this West African state-Ghana, varies in age, socio-economic status, education, geographical location and ethnic background too. Following the government's aim of 'health for all' currently, different categories of nurses are now being trained and employed in Ghana. What exists now even with the government's aim is that nursing in Ghana is seriously handicapped because the system lacks enough specialists in common health services for the work on hand. According to Maglacas (1986) nursing encompasses health promotion, prevention and rehabilitation. Nursing is something that is institutional, individual, and a proponent of self-care. The world Development Report (2004) express that except there is improvements to the human resources situation, stated health-related Millennium Development Goals cannot be attained. Reporting notes state that the problems of shortage of nurses are multiple. This exist especially in rural and remote areas. Mathauer and Imhoff (2006) states that especially for developing countries such as Ghana, adequate human resource management (HRM) and quality management too (QM) instruments used should be utilized to develop the work environment so that health workers like nurses and doctors who are motivated to meet their personal and organizational goals.

Conflict Prevention and Management

Just as we have mentioned earlier, as nurses, we do more of meeting people, communicating, offering emotional and psychological help. We work in a work chain which others. Nursing as a profession is totally based on collaborative relationships with colleagues and clients too. Conflicts can result from when two or more people view similar issues from two or multiple perspectives. Conflict here has to do with struggle in which a person may want to harass, neutralize, eliminate, and injure a rival. Most times, conflict is commonly perceived as a negative issue. But we can't hide from the fact that dealing with conflict can also bring positive outcomes for nurses, client and nurses too. As a nurse, if you fail to manage conflict effectively, it can hinder you from giving quality care to you client and it can also lead to abuse and violence (if it goes to the extreme). When we are relating to client care, when conflicts are not resolved, it continues to influence every aspect of the client care. It may surprise you that conflict is an inherent aspect of nursing. When you are providing professional services to clients, doesn't give the client the right to abuse you in any way. In fact, accepting abuses is far from your job description but resolving conflicts between you and your patient is very important. Nurses who have mastered the effective way to control antagonistic and passive-aggressive behaviors command respect from their clients and for their clients as well as their colleagues too. We would discuss some popular conflicts we experience as a nurse and how we can resolve them:

a. Nurse-Client conflict

The professional therapeutic relationship that exist between the nurse and the client serves as a foundation for the client's well-being and health. As a nurse, you should be ready to support the client to achieve the client's health goals. Nevertheless, unresolved conflict can hamper the attainment of these set goals. Conflict between a client and a nurse can escalate when one of all of the following happens to a client:

- When a client is totally intoxicated or under the influence of a substance

- When a client is being constrained. A very good example is if a client is prevented from smoking or any health-destructing habit.
- When a client is tensed, anxious, worried, disoriented or afraid.

Also, conflict between a nurse and a client can escalate when all or one of these happens:

- When a nurse labels, misunderstands or judges a client.
- If a nurse fails to listen, understand or respect the client's values, needs and also ethno cultural beliefs, it may result to real conflict of ideas.
- If a nurse speaks to a client using an improper tone of voice maybe speaking too loud, speaking so close or shouting.
- If as a nurse, you fail to provide enough information to satisfy the client or the client's family, conflict is in evitable.

How can this conflict be resolved as a nurse? Well I would offer you some points on that, but you should know that as a nurse, you are the one on the "pleasing" side of the table. You should not be too proud to apologize to your client when you are wrong and when you are not. The following are ways you can manage conflict, they can be also called conflict-management strategies. These strategies should be holistically and individually tailored to the specific needs of the client.

- As a nurse you should have a critical incident management plan.
- Be calm when relating to your client and enable them to share their concerns.
- At no point in time should you argue, criticize or judge any client.
- When you are handling the behavior development of a client, you should include the client's family and other health care team members.
- As a nurse, you should state it emphatically that abusive languages are not tolerated and you should not be guilty of the same offense.
- Maintain a physical gap between yourself and the client by stepping away from the client when necessary. Space boundaries must be obeyed.
- After you must have resolved a conflict, you should allow the situation to develop into a good plan of care

Conflict with colleagues

An indirect influence of nurse-patients conflict also affects the conflict between the nurse and colleagues. When poor relationships exist between members of the health care team, it negatively tells in the delivery of health care services. The conflict existing between a nurse and his/her colleagues can escalate if one or all of the following happens:

- If team members fail to support each other in realizing the client goals and responsibilities.
- If barriers to work together exist and there is no shared encouragement between each other.
- At times, colleagues are unintentionally or intentionally placed under serious conditions which may be beyond their capabilities.
- The fear of reprisal hampers the reporting of the misunderstanding or the conflict by staff.

As a nurse, you can manage conflict with colleagues using the following ways:

- Immediately when a conflict raises its hideous head, you should handle it and don't postpone its resolution.

- Make sure you concentrate on the result of the behavior that would lead to the conflict than the personality of the colleague.
- Cooperate with your colleagues to recognize the underlying cause of the conflict.

Workplace conflict

A proper definition of a healthy workplace is an environment where nurses can safely and properly recognize conflict and also implement the proper system for management. A workplace conflict has to do with the totality. An organizational conflict or workplace conflict can escalate due to the following reasons:

- If clarity of staff is not in place.
- When you have existing formal performance feedback processes, you don't affect the behaviors of the client or your colleagues.
- If the organizational policies are not properly communicated to staffs at all level, a conflict can escalate.
- When the managers and administrator bully or abuses others.

- When nurses and several healthcare professionals keep working at high stress or stressful conditions for a long period of time.
- In case, the workplace policy or culture supports under-reporting of events of conflicts.
- Workplace conflict can also escalate when there are intense organizational changes.
- If the staff perceive job insecurity, conflict can escalate.

Managing work place conflict can be done in the following ways:

- Instituting clear policies and punishments for those who break policies aimed at protecting the workplace from conflict and abuse.
- As a nurse, a system that promotes the denouncements of incidence of conflict in workplace should be put in place.
- Accessing the incidence of workplace conflict in routine can lead to corrective action. And this is a good way to manage workplace conflict.

Sexual Harassment

Every profession has its own risk and hazards. Sexual harassment exists as a psychological hazard which is faced by health workers at their workplace. The nature of nursing as a profession involves working "closely" with patients and staff members too. This may result to a physical and emotional attachment to those that are involved. Due to this, it is very possible and nurses could fall prey easily to those who take advantage of getting close to perpetrate the sex crime.

Sexual Harassment Defined

Two types of sexual harassment as covered by the Supreme Court by Title VII of the Civic Rights Act:

- *Quid pro quo:* Job security, advancement, or benefits are tied to sexual favors. This type includes unwelcome sexual advances, requests for sexual favors, or physical or verbal conduct of a sexual nature that are tied directly or implicitly to employment.
- Hostile work environment: Inappropriate behavior is so pervasive and severe that it permeates the workplace and interferes with the individual's ability to carry out the duties of the job.

The types of sexual harassment are as follows

1. Verbal (spoken or written): This has to do with offensive teasing, questioning, joking, etc. Making terms of endearment, such as "sweetie" "honey" or "hunk". The verbal sexual harassment can also showcase itself in: letters, inappropriate emails, and telephone calls, sensual and irrelevant comments about appearance or clothing. Spreading false news about someone's sexual life.
2. Non-verbal: showcasing sexual gestures like making hand signals, and eating in provocative manner can be sexual harassment. Giving gifts, looking inappropriately at someone's body part. Etc.
3. Visual: This has to do with sexual exposure "flashing" "mooning" offensive pictures, nude pictures, etc.

The best thing to do when you experience this, is to raise an alarm. Report to the authorities. If this persists, you have the right to report to the Nursing association. Health care institutions should have policies in place for dealing with outright sexual harassment from patients or client, and staffs too. This policy should be documented and reporting to the appropriate supervisor should be in place too. Surprisingly and sadly, females at the supervisory positions are speculated to be harassed more than females who are in subordinate positions. We should not take sexual harassment lightly because just as conflict and Gender discrimination can affect the staff, the patients and the healthcare institution in general.

www.ingramcontent.com/pod-product-compliance
Lightning Source LLC
Chambersburg PA
CBHW020910180526
45163CB00007B/2687